THE
BackPower
PROGRAM

THE BackPower PROGRAM

Dr. David Imrie
and
Dr. Lu Barbuto

First published in 1988 by
Stoddart Publishing Co. Limited
34 Lesmill Road
Toronto, Canada
M3B 2T6

Second printing — December 1988

CANADIAN CATALOGUING IN PUBLICATION DATA

Imrie, David
    Back power

1. Backache - Treatment.   2. Exercise therapy.
I. Barbuto, Lu   II. Title.

RD768.I57 1988   617'.56062   C88-094522-2

TEXT DESIGN: Brant Cowie/ArtPlus Limited

COVER PHOTOGRAPH: Peter Paterson

TYPE OUTPUT: Tony Gordon Ltd.

Printed and bound in the United States of America

The procedures and explanations given in this publication are based on research and consultation with medical and nursing authorities. To the best of our knowledge, these procedures and explanations reflect currently accepted medical practice; nevertheless, they can't be considered absolute and universal recommendations. For individual application, treatment suggestions must be considered in light of the individual's health, subject to a doctor's specific recommendations. The authors and the publisher disclaim responsibility for any adverse effects resulting directly or indirectly from the suggested procedures, from any undetected errors, or from the reader's misunderstanding of the text.

*To our patients from the past,
for teaching us what we know,
ensuring future patients
the best back health possible.*

Contents

THE BACK POWER STORY

Medicine and Chiropractic

The American Medical Association (AMA) is the most powerful medical organization in the world, with the second strongest lobby (after the aerospace industry) in the United States. It represents 225,000 medical doctors. The AMA has also historically been the worldwide "official" source of information on chiropractic methods and the chiropractic profession.

On August 27, 1987, a U.S. Federal Court in Chicago found that the AMA and various affiliated organizations, such as the American College of Radiology (ACR), had between 1966 and 1980 pursued an illegal conspiracy designed to contain and destroy the chiropractic profession.

On September 25, 1987, the Court delivered this injunction, or permanent restraining order, against the AMA:

> **The AMA, its officers, agents and employees, and all persons who act in active concert with any of them . . . are hereby permanently enjoined from restricting, regulating or impeding . . . the freedom of any AMA member or any institution or hospital to make an individual decision as to whether or not that AMA member, institution, or hospital, shall professionally associate with chiropractors, chiropractic students, or chiropractic institutions.**
>
> — Outcome of the Wilk case, an anti-trust action begun in 1976 and reported in the press nationwide on September 26, 1987.

We had followed the Wilk case with great interest and no little amazement. How could two professions of the healing arts — both dedicated to serving humanity by alleviating suffering — end up in a court of law?

This traditional enmity was counter to our own experience: for more than a decade, we had been working together to improve our approach to humankind's oldest enemy: *back pain*. By bringing our professions *together*, we had developed an effective program, called Back Power, which is the subject of this book. But before we tell you what the Back Power program can do for you, we'll each explain how it happened that a medical doctor and a chiropractor began such a collaboration.

David Imrie, M.D. —

A Physician Looks at Backs

O f all the problems encountered by the occupational health physician, there is none greater than that of the problem back. It affects more people over longer periods of time than any other condition and it is unsurpassed for testing the patience of both doctors trying to diagnose, manage, and treat the problem and sufferers trying to recover from it. A complex, costly problem, the impact of back pain on individuals is in the same league as heart disease, cancer, and respiratory illnesses.

When I began to practice in the late 1960s, conventional wisdom stated that back problems resulted from damage or injury caused by excessive forces: "lifting the wrong way," slipping, or falling — or else were caused by internal disease that became externally manifested by back pain. I had been trained accordingly. As an occupational health physician, I was using a neuro-orthopedic assessment designed to determine whether disease was present, whether there was injury and structural damage, and whether surgical intervention was required.

As I examined patient after patient with low back pain, I was amazed at the relatively small number for whom I could make a definite diagnosis where specific medical or surgical intervention was indicated. Fortunately, most people recover from their bout of back pain, regardless of the type of treatment applied — but that wasn't good enough for me. Being a young, university-hospital-trained physician with a firm basis in science, I was curious to know more about a condition where conventional scientific methods seemed to produce so few positive findings. My scientific training also rebelled at the then-accepted hypothesis that minor tears to the discs were the source of pain in the large number of patients for whom there were no tangible findings. These tears, it was said, were too minute to be detected by conventional means. This conclusion impressed me as being not science but pseudo-science, an unproven hypothesis.

My duties as an occupational physician included certifying people as fit for work after they had recovered from a back injury and, for new employees, fit for work on preplacement assessment. Using traditional methods of examination on these apparently healthy and fit patients produced virtually no positive clinical findings. Yet the absence of findings in no way guaranteed that either group could perform without a new or recurrent back problem for one week, six weeks, six months, or six years. Clearly, my clinical experience began to challenge conventional wisdom about the examination and treatment of low backs.

What about Chiropractors?

I soon encountered another reality: in the companies that I served, many workers with back and other musculoskeletal problems had been seeing chiropractors. Not only did these workers seem pleased with the results, they were also prepared to go back for chiropractic treatment when necessary. I also noted that many were at first reluctant to tell me they had consulted a chiropractor, thinking this revelation would make me angry or create negative feelings. As I came to realize how much faith many people had in their chiropractors, I concluded that these health professionals must have something to offer. I was determined to find out what it was. At the same time, I reviewed in my mind those negative opinions about chiropractors that I had heard from my own profession. There were basically four concerns.

Chiropractors have a different theory of disease vs. health. Physicians basically look at health as the absence of disease, with disease defined as the encroachment of pathological processes on a healthy body. The purpose of the medical approach is thus to diagnose and eradicate the causes of this disease. Chiropractors emphasize the active pursuit of health, believing that it can be improved not only by restoring spinal function but by improving the habits of life-style: good diet, fresh air, exercise, sleeping and working practices. In short, chiropractic pioneered the holistic approach to health care.

Chiropractic treatment is empirically based. While medicine looks at disease from the organic pathological viewpoint — its treatments including drugs and/or surgery — chiropractic is a drugless, nonsurgical approach. Chiropractic's primary focus on disease is on structure — its effect on the nervous system and, hence, on the patient's health.

Chiropractic training is inadequate, especially for examination. Physicians accuse chiropractors of sometimes failing to diagnose disease — with disastrous consequences — and of treating, by means of manual adjustment, conditions that physicians believe can be treated properly only by medical means. (I later found out that chiropractic training in the basic sciences is virtually the same as that leading to the M.D. degree — with the exception of pharmacology. Like other primary-care practitioners, chiropracters are trained to recognize when medical or surgical intervention is required for a condition.)

Chiropractors make excessive use of X-rays. Physicians, looking for structural disease or trauma, usually require three to five static X-ray views to elucidate the problem. Chiropractors sometimes require more views to make their diagnoses. That is because they study function and dynamic motion throughout the spine to determine what is normal and what is abnormal.

But with these concerns came a reminder of the adage that "the conservatism of the medical profession is its greatest strength . . . but also can be its greatest weakness." I may have had fears about investigating chiropractic methods, but I was also determined to know more about them.

First, I simply wanted to do a better job of helping my patients with spinal problems. I had become convinced by what so many of them were telling me: their chiropractors' results were superior to my own!

Second, for purely business reasons in my occupational practice I knew that I must develop better answers for this most common, costly, and frustrating problem. I felt I must learn what chiropractors had to offer.

Third, I was drawn by curiosity: just what did these chiropractors do that created great faith and positive feelings among many members of the general public but continued to elicit hostility or apathy from my own profession?

So it was that I mustered my courage and phoned the dean of the Canadian Memorial Chiropractic College to arrange for a meeting with one of its residents. I wanted to learn what the chiropractic approach was all about. That was how Lu Barbuto and I met. Step by step, we began to work together for a more satisfactory approach to our patients' problems.

Lu Barbuto, D.C. —

Personal experience of back injury from playing football as a high school junior introduced me to North America's third largest health profession, chiropractic.

Conventional medical examination and X-rays had shown no pathology in my back, yet I continued to experience pain. After a summer of therapy, I returned to my senior year and attempted to pursue my sports activities. When my back pain persisted, my wrestling coach, an excellent athlete and personal mentor, recommended that I see a chiropractor. At 16, I knew little about the chiropractic profession or methods and went to my first appointment with some serious reservations.

The chiropractic management of my problem proved successful. I was impressed by the conservative and structural approach to health care, and soon decided to make chiropractic my career.

When David Imrie approached me about learning more about chiropractic methods and how chiropractors could assist him in his occupational practice, I thought back to my first two weeks of chiropractic care. They had given me a unique opportunity to experience and compare the main features of the chiropractic approach to health care with the medical approach. The bottom line was that the hi-tech sophistication of the latter had done nothing for me. The chiropractic low-tech approach had helped.

In terms of low back problems, what I had to contribute was a focus on the relationship of the whole body to the spine and the musculoskeletal system. This would be a new perspective for an M.D. trained in the medical sciences.

A Chiropractor Looks at Backs

Chiropractic may be defined as the study of health problems and disease from a structural point of view, with special consideration given to the mechanics of the spine and its relationship to the nervous system.

My six years of chiropractic study taught me to explore and challenge many accepted concepts of health and disease. Conventional medicine as we know it today adheres to Western philosophy based on the concept of preventing, inhibiting and curing disease through the use of drugs and surgery. It is centered around institutions such as hospitals that offer an array of technological wizardry, specialists, and ancillary services, with its gate-keepers the members of one profession. Despite medicine's enormous technological advances and great successes, the use of health-care services has continued to increase, the side effects from treatment are sometimes costing more than the actual treatment of the illness itself, and there seems to be no end to the rise in health-care costs.

So it was with doubts of my own that I began a decade ago to work with David Imrie. During those years, we've influenced each other in terms of our perspective on health and disease, exchanging and supplementing viewpoints. We've come to the conclusion that health cannot be the exclusive domain of one profession. Rather, by challenging current concepts and taking an interdisciplinary approach to the problems associated with the diagnosis, treatment, and management of back pain, we've arrived at our mutual goal: helping you to help yourself be the best you can be, *whether or not you've ever experienced back pain*. That is the subject of this book. We call it Back Power.

1

The Back Power Story

Medicine was in the ascendancy in the late 1960s, unlocking the mysteries of the cell and DNA, developing powerful antibiotics, perfecting methods of organ transplant, substituting artificial parts for diseased ones. It was a time of high-tech revolution.

Yet 125 or so years before, clusters of symptoms for the first time had been put together to make medical diagnoses of specific diseases; until then, each symptom had been treated on its own merit. Right up to the mid-1800s, blood-letting was used to treat any condition that involved a fever. And it was only as recently as 1847 that Ignaz Semmelweis, a Hungarian physician and obstetrician, realized the importance of sterilizing surgical instruments and properly disinfecting the hands before examining patients.

With the recognition that conditions such as fever and pain were actually symptoms of organic disease and that the disease in turn was caused by infective agents, came the recognition that there were specific treatments for each disease. As modern medicine evolved, its goals expanded. Today we seek not only to limit the natural history of a disease (the course a disease takes if left untreated) but to improve lifespan and increase the quality of life.

Modern Medicine

Who were the parents of modern medicine as we know it? Virchow, the great pathologist, was the first to recognize abnormalities in organs and tissues. He defined specific diseases, which he understood to be revealed by specific symptoms and tests. His gathering of these clusters or constellations of signs and symptoms to identify disease is recognized as the major advance that ushered in the "golden age of medicine." Virchow was followed by Pasteur, who studied germs and their relationship to disease and invented pasteurization; by Pierre and Marie Curie, who at the turn of the century discovered the effects of X-rays; by Sir Alexander Fleming, who discovered penicillin; and by Sir Frederick Banting and Charles Best, who co-developed insulin for the treatment of diabetes.

By the second World War, medicine was well on its way to being integrated into the scientific age. People were starting to live longer and better. But most of the credit was given to the new technologies that medicine was devising, and few people realized then that the major health enhancement in our society had come not from the marvels of high-tech *treatment* of disease but from low-tech, behind-the-scenes *prevention*. Water purification, sewage treatment, and mass immunization have contributed more to quality and length of life than all antibiotic treatments combined.

In 1962, the Nobel Prize in medicine and physiology was awarded to Francis Crick, Maurice Wilkins, and James D. Watson for their discovery of the double helix of DNA — the start of genetic research, which delves into the structural code of life itself. Today we are actually engineering artificial genes and genetic products that have the promise of reshaping our lives.

Many people, while accepting these high-tech advances in medicine, still yearn for the days of the caring health professional who practiced the healing art as such. This letter, reprinted from a medical journal, describes a time that actually wasn't long ago:

In 1935 my little black bag contained many drugs that most doctors trained in the past quarter of a century have not heard of, or at least not in a therapeutic context: the expectorants ammonium chloride and ipecac; the "alternatives" nux vomica and arsenic, used in tonics; the various bromide salts, each with a supposedly different function; and tincture valerian, a sedative, particularly useful in psychoneurosis. These were the drugs that a doctor gave to a patient with the expectation, on the part of both, that they had curative or at least restorative properties.

Today the administration of those drugs by a physician might be considered quackery. As used in patent medicines now, they are spoken of with deprecation. Yet 50 years ago the recovery of patients from many diseases was ascribed to these chemicals.

Today we bemoan the loss of the art of medicine. Was this not the act of instilling in the patient faith in the doctor and what he or she prescribed? In other words, was not the practice of medicine before the so-called miracle drugs faith healing? Faith in the doctor stimulated or strengthened the *vis medicatrix naturae*, the natural defensive and healing power, and possibly the immune system in particular.·

Faith in doctors was, I believe, much greater then than it is now. I think of an episode involving my father, a physician: In 1912 he was on a train bound for Toronto from Red Deer, Alberta. At Regina he was given a telegram that read: 'My wife dangerously ill with pneumonia. We need you.' My father returned to Red Deer on the next train and sat with the patient until she had her crisis. It is difficult to believe that such faith had little to do with her recovery.

— W.B. Parsons, M.D. Sylvan Lake, Alberta (*CMA Journal*, vol. 133, Oct. 1, 1985)

David Imrie, M.D. —

High Tech vs. Low Tech

On graduating from medical school in 1968, I decided to enter family practice for a few years to get a sound clinical base before specializing — in ophthalmology, I thought then. Here, I began to deal with the realities of ordinary people's diseases and to realize how different they were from the skewed sample of diseases seen in a university teaching hospital. I had been well trained in the scientific approach to disease: chief complaint; history of past and present illness; complete examination; tests; forming a differential diagnosis; final diagnosis or cause; treatment; prognosis. I knew how to deliver a baby, take out an appendix, operate on tonsils, and deal with an acute heart attack. But I had little knowledge of how to deal with aches and sprains, colds, counseling for simple problems such as a baby refusing its milk or medication, advising elderly patients on specific concerns, or working with patients suffering mentally or socially. These were low-tech problems, requiring a low-tech approach, and my training was wanting.

My first few years in practice found me dealing with a high incidence of disease, and then I found myself working mainly with chronic and degenerative problems and conditions that could be improved or limited only through changes in a patient's life-style or behavior. It was not a treatment situation, but one of prevention in some cases and management in others. More often than not, high-technology answers just didn't enter the picture.

Preventive Health Care: The Life-Style Message.

This was a time of great ferment in medical care. It was finally dawning on politicians and administrators that high-tech medicine with its infinitely expanding capabilities was about to clash with the economic realities of affordability. An increasingly large percentage of the gross national product was being consumed by medical treatments and cures. There was no end in sight for the annual escalation in costs to keep people healthy.

But at the same time there was an obvious shift in the types of disease afflicting people in this second half of our century. Behavior and life-style began to be recognized as having tremendous influence not only on the *kinds* of disease that people had, but on the early manifestations. The association between cigarette smoking and lung cancer even then was well documented, though disputed by many. And the significant increase in heart disease, stroke, and other cardiovascular problems was beginning to be attributed to dietary excesses — particularly excess fat and cholesterol — and lack of fitness. Back pain, arthritis, ulcers, asthma, bronchitis, and many other conditions had strong life-style connections.

The concern about defining health as the absence of disease or sickness, the tremendous cost escalation, the emerging association of life-style, behavior, and disease — all these factors had come under the scrutiny of Marc Lalonde, then Canada's health minister. In a statement entitled *A New Perspective on the Health of Canadians*, he put forward the view that health is influenced by a broad range of factors, including everything that contributes to life-style: our physical, social, and work environments. He advocated a new emphasis on preventive health care, focusing on changing those factors with negative or harmful consequences. This was a message that excited me with its possibilities.

The Low-Tech Route to the Boston Marathon

Not far from my own clinic in the early 1970s, Dr. Terry Kavanagh was revolutionizing the care of patients recovering from heart problems. A rehabilitation specialist, Dr. Kavanagh directly opposed the conventions of the day with his low-tech approach.

Traditionally, individuals who had suffered heart attacks were advised to avoid all activity and exertion thereafter — effectively resting for the balance of their lives. But Dr. Kavanagh's patients, once their hearts had healed sufficiently, went on a diet and graded exercise regimen. The results were amazing. These people could function significantly better than they had before their heart attacks. One group actually completed the Boston Marathon! At 26+ miles, a marathon is something that relatively few people ever even *attempt* in a lifetime, let alone complete. This group didn't compete with the winners, but they did finish without suffering any problems. (If this feat has been eclipsed in the past few years by a heart transplant patient who also completed a marathon run, its significance remains undiminished.)

I became interested in what Dr. Kavanagh had achieved with his patients and began to incorporate into my own practice his philosophy of life-style/behavior modification. As I did, I began to see that many of the sicknesses that we considered as diseases, to be *diagnosed* and treated, were in reality conditions that could be *managed* better by the combination of treatment and long-term life-style improvement. This approach assumed my best efforts as a health professional and the patient's active participation and cooperation.

The World Health Organization has stated that health is not just the absence of disease but a resource for everyday living: "The extent to which an individual or group is able on the one hand to realize aspirations and satisfy needs and on the other hand, to change or cope with the environment." Health, in other words, is best defined by *functional capacity* — the ability to *live* life, to work hard and to play hard.

The Hidden Epidemic

As well as practicing family medicine, early in my career I took over the occupational/medical practice that had been founded 30 years earlier by Dr. Wilf Auger. Said to be the oldest occupational health clinic in Canada, it served a number of industries.

Now I began to round out my training as I saw evidence of the influences of work and work environments on individuals' health. There were the obvious influences: high noise levels in work areas over many years, creating occupational deafness; people working with epoxies and suffering from dermatitis or eczema; isocyanates at work, causing occupational asthma.

What interested me most, however, was what I like to call the hidden epidemic: people with low back, neck, and other musculoskeletal disorders. These cases accounted by far for the majority of problems that I saw in my occupational practice.

When someone came to me complaining of this type of pain, my approach was to diagnose the cause and to get the patient pain-free again. The problem was that no matter how well I examined the back, no matter how many tests and X-rays I had done, no matter how many specialists I referred the patient to, I was rarely able to define a specific illness that could be given a specific treatment and would have a specific prognosis with a confident outcome in the future. Low back problems were much more frustrating to deal with than broken legs, ruptured appendices, or heart attacks because they seemed to be so imprecise, their causes so difficult to trace, and their outcome and treatment so unpredictable. In addition, it seemed that once the problems hit, they would not only recur throughout a worker's career but would become worse, of longer duration, and harder to deal with as each new bout developed.

It was doubly frustrating to try to find some weakness in the low back that would respond to any kind of preventive action. Here was a dilemma. The traditional symptom/diagnosis approach was not working. If a high-tech approach was sought, it could mean something as extreme as disc transplants. I thought again about Dr. Kavanagh and realized that, just maybe, a low-tech, commonsense approach to low back problems could provide some answers.

The Muscle Factor

At this point, bearing in mind that conventional low back X-rays were such poor indicators of future risk, I turned my attention to muscles. I clearly remember the day I examined Harry, a 45-year-old mechanic who had injured his back at work and was having recurrent problems. He was seated across from me in my office, looking unfit and overweight. As I pondered his problem, I was reminded of my dad.

Dad was a tool and diemaker, and at 45 he had injured his back at work. Like Harry, he suffered numerous recurrences of back pain throughout his career, though his problem had been complicated by an accident. My father visited family doctors, was referred to a world-renowned orthopedic specialist, and went through various tests — all to no avail. Medication, physiotherapy, and chiropractic treatments helped somewhat, but the problem persisted relentlessly. Night after night he slept on the floor and was often irritable from his pain and loss of sleep. He never missed a day of work, however.

I'll never forget the night Dad announced at the supper table that he'd given up on remedies and treatments. He was going down to the

YMCA, he said, and if it killed him he would get back into shape. Soon an amazing thing happened: as he exercised and began to improve his fitness, reducing his weight as well, he found that his back pain was not so severe. He continued to exercise, and eventually the pain disappeared to the extent that he never suffered from it again during his long life.

As I looked at my mechanic friend, I realized that I really knew very little that was specific about back fitness. Referring to my medical textbooks, I was surprised to find almost nothing about how to deal with weak or strained muscles or muscle imbalance. I thought then of the very short medical school course on physical therapy and muscles. It had been placed during the spring term . . . just around spring fever time.

Developing a Program

I had one great advantage. My sister Janet was a trained physiotherapist who, at the start of my occupational practice, had worked for several years with an orthopedic surgeon under the auspices of the Canadian Arthritic Society. Jan had developed an early back care program called "Support Your Local Back." It was an education program designed to help sufferers become involved in managing their low back problems, and had been well received.

Jan and I began to work with groups, teaching back education. We also continued working one-to-one with individual low back sufferers. It became apparent that most people lacked health knowledge and information about the basics of anatomy as well as how to sit, stand, and walk correctly. We realized too that knowledge must be linked to capability — you can't teach the rules of football and then expect the person to play. The individual's commitment and effort are essential.

We had another major challenge to contend with, which we christened Imrie's Law: *a person's interest in back pain varies inversely with the length of time since the last pain experience.* In other words, when the back pain settles down, most people feel they are fit again. They are not convinced of the need for that extra effort to keep the back fit and functioning.

Certain that a simple and persuasive demonstration was needed to get people's attention and focus it on the state of their backs — even when pain-free — we set about to find a test that could begin to define low back dysfunction.

The Kraus Connection   About 15 years earlier, a New York City specialist, Dr. Hans Kraus, had also recognized the need for such tests. Concerned with fitness and health as they related to the low back, Dr. Kraus had developed Kraus-Weber tests, which were incorporated into a special back care/fitness program designed by the YM/YWCA (*The Y's Way to a Healthy Back*).

In an occupational setting, Jan and I eagerly applied the six Kraus-Weber tests, which had been designed to help individuals define their functions of strength and capability. We found with experience, however, that these tests frequently gave people a false sense of security. In too many instances, our occupational patients who had suffered back pain in the past and would suffer again in the future, passed the tests easily. We concluded that the idea of the tests, although basically good, needed updating and further refinement.

In making these refinements, we stressed the functions of the low back: (1) movement and flexibility; and (2) the need to stabilize the back in lifting and weight-bearing and in order to protect the spinal column from injury. Our tests would be designed to measure the strength of the four types of supporting trunk muscles: stomach, back, sling, and lateral muscles. From this basic premise, we developed the National Back Fitness Test. This test would not only help us to define a weak back but would guide us as we proceeded to recondition the back muscles to an individual's personal best.

The Failure Factor   At first we used an exercise program based on a flexion routine. This meant that we gave a great deal of attention to strengthening the stomach muscles as well as having people incorporate the pelvic tilt in their exercise program. The pelvic tilt is a type of exercise that teaches people coordination of the trunk in lifting and emphasizes good balance.

This routine worked successfully with a large number of people, but there was a fairly consistent minority that did not do well at all with our type of approach, and a small, persistent group that did worse: their back pain was aggravated.

We realized then — and have often confirmed since — that we learn most from our failures. Failures teach us more than our successes. In this case, what was most interesting about the group that did not benefit from the flexion routine was that they tended to be quite athletic people who appeared to be in good shape. They were usually thin, seemingly fit and healthy, yet they still complained of back problems.

Out of this failure came the next lesson in the evolution of our program: that muscle strength is a product of balanced muscle length, which is achieved through exercise and flexibility. It was a lesson to be underlined by personal experience.

Stretching Since leaving medical school, I had played a regular game of ice hockey every Thursday night, summer or winter, with a group of "oldtimers." The game was important to my own fitness routine and it helped me let off the steam accumulated from the demands of a heavy medical practice.

During one game I "pulled" a groin muscle. This is a common injury in ice hockey, and it seemed minor enough at the time. Unfortunately for my game, it became persistent: each time I thought it had eased I would start to skate again and, with very little effort exerted, re-injure the muscle. I began to think I'd have to give up my career as an oldtimer.

Then I was fortunate enough to meet Gord Stewart, a well-known fitness expert and author. Gord's expertise came from both his personal training and his own participation in the decathlon, that most grueling of Olympic events.

On hearing about my problem, Gord sat me down on the floor to show me a stretch/flexibility exercise. As I got in position to do the exercise, I noticed at once that the injured muscle had become much shorter and tighter than the healthy one. When I injured the muscle originally, it had contracted and gone into spasm; now, although the pain and spasm were gone, the muscle had been left short and weak. It was thus highly susceptible to recurrent injury.

It was a very short step from that realization to the conclusion that the same process might well be at work in people with low back problems. I was reminded of the Blix curve muscle experiment from my pre-med years. This experiment illustrated that the length and power of a muscle are interrelated — that muscles which are "musclebound" and tight could be weak and needed to be stretched to their optimal working length.

When we began to incorporate flexibility and extension exercises into our back program, we found that as a result our group of previously poor performers mostly showed a marked improvement.

So a cornerstone of the Back Power program was laid: a test of strength and flexibility of each of the four types of trunk muscles, followed by an exercise program dictated by personal test results.

Still there was more to learn, and it was at this point that I decided to investigate chiropractic methods. My association with Lu Barbuto would result in another cornerstone for Back Power.

Lu Barbuto, D.C. —

An Emphasis on Function

Historically, the chiropractic approach to treatment was first mentioned as an accepted form of therapy by Hippocrates in ancient Greece; the word "chiropractic" is from the Greek and means "treatment by hand." In contemporary terms, Canadian-born Daniel David Palmer is regarded as the founder of modern chiropractic, in 1895.

The chiropractic model is in most ways the essence of low technology. Handing the responsibility of health care back to the individual, it proclaims that the body has a natural ability to fight disease and achieve stable health. My training had introduced me to the holistic approach to health care before it became fashionable in North America.

Today, chiropractors have the most extensive education and training to carry out spinal manual therapy — "manipulation" — properly and safely. With our emphasis on *function* rather than *structure*, we look for functional abnormality in a patient's spine; the medical practitioner looks for structural abnormality.

As I started to work with David at his clinic, we realized that even our basic terminology differed greatly. But I agreed to work with him two half-days weekly, examining together the most chronic, difficult backs. We would then compare notes. David quickly realized the importance of functional spinal movements and applied himself to learning manual examination techniques and diagnosis.

Although the road looked a bit long, it also appeared promising. What we didn't realize at first, however, was just how deeply rooted were our different perspectives: mine in the function of joints plus the efficacy of restoring movement to fixed joints; David's in the importance of the muscular support to the low back and the importance of strength and flexibility through muscle balance. Although we were tolerant of each other's viewpoints, we often tended to rely on the approach that each of us knew best.

Bridging the Gap

At the start of our collaboration, we attended several seminars on the topic of manipulation. David seemed somewhat surprised to see not only chiropractors and osteopaths, but also physicians who were also interested in adjustment/mobilization.

Gradually, David began to appreciate the importance of normal function in the movement of joints and its relationship not only to the relieving of pain but to the *preventing* of dysfunction and a predisposition toward weakness and pain. He came to realize the significance not only of the gross movements of the back but of the movements of each spinal segment.

My training meant that I could show David how to recognize that a fixation at one level of the spine could cause excessive movement, pain, and instability at adjacent levels — that problems at one level would influence joints at other levels, causing additional problems, pain, and even disease. Alongside Imrie's Law, I introduced Barbuto's Warning: *Think function, not pain — or expect problems again.*

Finally we came to realize that the whole approach to the back is much more sound with a united point of view. There is a place for muscles, and equally there is a place for joint function. The ultimate challenge, we agreed, was to determine *who needs what form of treatment* for low back pain, prevention, and care.

Back Power: All in All

Perhaps the most important influence on the Back Power program is that of the workers we see in our occupational clinic. We listen to them and we learn from them. They know their jobs better than we ever could. They also know their pain and their pain experience better than we could ever understand. By listening to them, we have learned what works and what does not. We're prepared to share that information with you.

The Back Power program is not just a program of *treatment*; it's a program for *management* of back problems. Back Power isn't seeking a cure; it's a program of control. In Back Power, we don't look just at *back pain*; we also realize the importance of *painless dysfunction*, which can lead to pain, weakness, and disability. Nor do we look at prevention only; our concern, rather, is a form of prevention that will, if back pain does come, link with the treatment and ultimate management of the problem.

Back Power is not a health-professional-centered program. Rather it is a program which offers the best that health professionals can provide. At the same time, it expects the best that individuals can offer to minimize and manage their problem.

Back Power is not the result of one perspective on a problem but the assimilation of many points of view — physician, chiropractor, physiotherapist, fitness expert, and patient. The key to Back Power is a philosophy of balance: balance of muscles and joints; balance of health science and art; balance of effort from practitioner and patient; balance of treatment and prevention; balance between chiropractor and physician.

And the secret of it all is to identify the *imbalance* — to identify *who needs what*.

GETTING TO KNOW YOUR BACK: FUNCTION AND DYSFUNCTION

2

Back Pain: Cause and Effect

P ain is perhaps the most frequent and certainly the most alarming manifestation of disease in our bodies: chest pain that is caused by coronary artery disease; renal colic, the pain associated with kidney stones; the acute abdominal pain of appendicitis. In modern societies, the problem of pain generates two questions: what is causing the pain, and how do I get relief from it?

The usual approach to pain is making a diagnosis of disease and then treating the disease to remove the cause of the pain, at the same time giving the patient relief from discomfort. With renal colic, for instance, after the diagnosis is made and steps taken to remove the kidney stone, treatment of the pain is appropriate.

As we shall see, traditionally most approaches to spinal-related disorders have been directed toward "quick fixes" for symptomatic pain relief rather than aimed at making a meaningful diagnosis and correcting the underlying mechanical problems that are causing the pain.

Evaluating Pain

T he practical management of pain and a more fundamental approach to the various problems relating to the experience of pain are greatly hampered by our inability to objectively assess or measure its nature and intensity. In evaluating pain, we are entirely dependent on our patients' statements and behavior as well as on our interpretation of the symptoms they show or describe. Many patients express their frustration in trying to convey the intensity of their pain experience with remarks such as, "Doctor, you can't see inside my head, you cannot feel just how bad this pain is."

There is little doubt that low back pain will affect the quality of life for a majority of people in contemporary society at some time in their lives. In addition, many people today attach exaggerated importance to the slightest irritation of their sensitivity, trying much more than their ancestors to eliminate even the most trivial pain. Think back through the centuries. Backache, toothache, headache, gouty aches and the like have existed for thousands of years. And although natural herbs and plant medicines as well as alcohol and some narcotics have long been available to blunt the malevolent intruder, no society before ours has had access to such a broad range of analgesics and pain-relieving, mood-altering drugs or, it follows, has had such inclination to use these with wild abandon. Today, the wide range of over-the-counter and prescribed medications for pain vie only with tranquilizers as the most commonly used medications in our society.

Has the nature of pain changed through the centuries to demand such an overwhelming response? Has our capacity or willingness to withstand discomfort altered proportionately to our ready access to artificial "feeling good"? Has our pursuit of personal happiness and comfort caused unrealistic expectations and demands?

This perspective has, in part, misled or misdirected our approach to the treatment of spinal-related disorders: we focus on pain rather than on functional changes. The quality and intensity of musculoskeletal pain are extremely difficult for patients to convey, as are the nature and degree of stress produced by pain. Yet the behavior of pain, when related to intensity, time, posture, and movement, can provide a sound basis for assessment.

Pain Is Important

To those of us interested in the study of human ailments, it is scarcely necessary to emphasize the value of pain as a symptom. Pain is an unpleasant sensory experience distinct from other sensory experiences, such as touch, warmth, and cold. Pain gives information about states of the body but, unlike other sensations, not about the nature of the stimulus. Pain cannot be defined in words that would mean anything to someone who has not experienced it. It is a subjective affair, in short, and when it relates to the musculoskeletal system, pain may result from: fatigued muscles, faulty posture, dysfunction in spinal dynamics, asymmetrical muscle loading, injury or trauma, muscle spasm, ligament strain, or spinal disease — all of which we'll explain in detail.

Pain signals actual or impending tissue damage, and a knowledge of how spinal pain can arise and of how it is transmitted and interpreted in the nervous system is essential to both practitioner and patient. In recent years, detailed principles in the sciences of neurohistology and neurophysiology (sciences of the cells and function of the nervous system) have been clearly set out. As a result, it is now easier to provide a more orderly account of the clinical significance of spinal pain states. For one thing is certain: *spinal pain is not normal. It must be assessed, understood, and dealt with.*

How Pain Is Transmitted to the Brain

Figure 2.1 depicts the way in which pain is transmitted to the brain. Essentially pain is interpreted by *afferent* nerve fibers. (Afferent nerves are incoming; in this case, they transmit painful stimuli *to* the brain. *Efferent* nerves lead away from the brain.) Our pain receptors are located in the skin, in deeper tissue such as muscles and *fascia* (tissue connecting and surrounding the organs), and in internal organs.

FIG. 2.1 HOW PAIN IS TRANSMITTED TO THE BRAIN

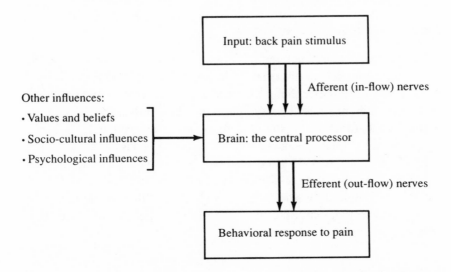

When an impulse is produced by stimulation of a pain receptor, it enters the spinal cord, through which it ascends to the brain. There, the impulse is localized and interpreted by the various portions of the brain in terms of its previous painful experience. The skin, for example, is touched many times, meaning that the sensory portion of the brain is so frequently programmed with this familiar image that it can localize stimuli from the skin with great precision. We can pinpoint pain anywhere on the skin. Impulses from deeper structures such as ligaments of the spine reach consciousness less often and are therefore less familiar to the brain.

Pain Is Subjective

The perception of any sensation depends not just on the appropriate receptor cells in skin, muscle, joint, or organ and the integrity of the peripheral nerve and spinal cord pathways, but on complex connections within the brain that may be influenced by the thoughts and emotions of the individual.

So it is that all sensation, including pain, is subjective. Each individual has a personal "perceptual scope" that is unique and can be known to others solely by the individual's ability to describe it. That description involves a series of complex interactions that merge the psychological, physiological, socio-cultural, and clinical aspects of pain.

Pain Is a Symptom, Not a Disease

For just more than one hundred years, physicians have been using the "medical model" to discover the cause of disease. This is the method of interviewing and examining the patient in an attempt to find the cause of the symptom reported. This symptom may be a rash, some difficulty in normal bodily function, or pain. It is important to understand that pain is a *symptom*, not a disease in itself. When we come to consider back pain, it is also important to understand that only sometimes does the medical model lead to a diagnosis of disease; more often, it does not.

Let's look first at the structure of the back and then at the nature of those diseases that can affect it — the diseases that can produce back pain as a *symptom*.

Structure of the Back

The human spinal column is the center of postural control, the framework in our effort to retain upright posture against the force of gravity. It is built to provide a maximum degree of stability and at the same time allow a maximum of flexibility. On the one hand, it is a pillar of support, and on the other it can be likened to beads (vertebrae) strung together.

The two seemingly incompatible functions of support (inflexibility) and movement (flexibility) are opposite ends of a spectrum of movement, and this fact is one reason the spine is so vulnerable to injury. It is only through ligamentous and muscular support that the two functions can be carried out.

The head is supported upon the seven *cervical vertebrae* that make up the neck. The *thoracic vertebrae* are twelve in number, and serve as the anchoring system for the ribs. The lower back comprises five *lumbar vertebrae*, which lie between the chest and the pelvis. The base of the spine is composed of the *sacrum* and the *coccyx*, which form the midback of the pelvic cavity (see figure 2.2).

FIG. 2.2 SPINAL (VERTEBRAL) COLUMN

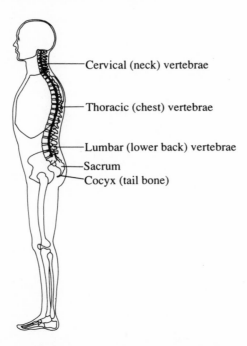

Cervical (neck) vertebrae

Thoracic (chest) vertebrae

Lumbar (lower back) vertebrae

Sacrum

Cocyx (tail bone)

The spinal column is often compared to a rod formed of a series of spools (vertebrae) placed one upon the other. Down through the holes of the spools runs the spinal cord, and out through the openings between the vertebrae pass the spinal nerves. In the space between the vertebrae lies a spongy shock absorber referred to as the *intervertebral disc*. The purpose of the discs is to provide the spinal column with shape and resiliency, permitting it to transmit loads by compressing, then springing back into shape to restore the vertebrae to their original position when weight-bearing is over.

When viewed from the side, the spinal column presents three gentle curvatures, forward and backward (see figure 2.3). They are referred to as *cervical lordosis, thoracic kyphosis*, and *lumbar lordosis*. All three curves must meet in the midline center of gravity to balance the weight distribution of the whole curve and to counter the eccentric loading of each curve. On the one hand, gentle curves render strength to the spinal column. On the other, as curves increase in deviation from the center-of-gravity line or as posture becomes abnormal and exaggerated, the spine becomes weaker and more vulnerable to stress, strain, and injury.

FIG. 2.3 **NORMAL SPINAL CURVES**

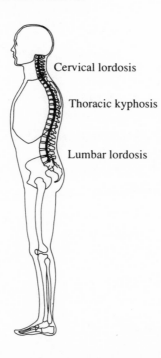

Cervical lordosis

Thoracic kyphosis

Lumbar lordosis

One-quarter of the adult spine is composed of disc material, with the remaining three-quarters consisting of bony vertebrae. Figure 2.4 shows what the vertebrae look like and how they are linked together.

FIG. 2.4 BUILDING BLOCKS OF THE SPINAL COLUMN

A

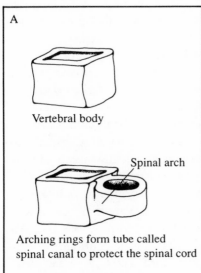

Vertebral body

Spinal arch

Arching rings form tube called
spinal canal to protect the spinal cord

B

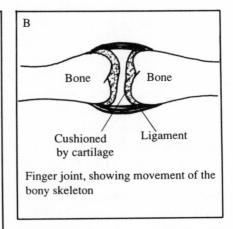

Bone   Bone

Cushioned   Ligament
by cartilage

Finger joint, showing movement of the
bony skeleton

C

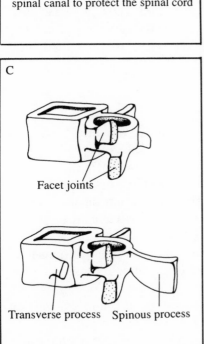

Facet joints

Transverse process   Spinous process

D

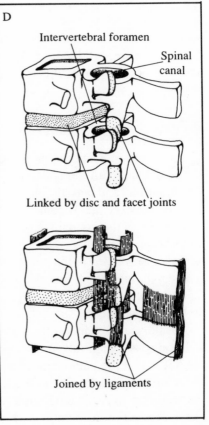

Intervertebral foramen

Spinal
canal

Linked by disc and facet joints

Joined by ligaments

The front or thicker part of each vertebra, which is very strong, is called the *vertebral body*; at the back of the vertebrae are the *facet joints*, linked to the solid front part by *arching rings* (A). The facet joints function to permit movement and flexibility in the spine. Similar to the finger joints (B), they consist of two bones covered by articular cartilage, which gives a spongy, shock-absorbing resiliency to the joint, and are joined together by ligaments. The lining of the joint is enclosed with *synovial membrane*, which produces fluid to fill the joint space for further shock-absorbing capacity.

The bony protrusions at the side of the vertebrae are called *transverse processes* and are for the attachment of muscles; at the back are *spinous* processes, to which muscles and ligaments are attached (C). Each vertebral body is separated from the next in front by the spongy disc and is linked behind by two facet joints at each level.

The whole column is linked by a series of strong fibrous cords (ligaments) joining all the bones together at various positions (D). All the vertebrae fit together neatly to form that rod or continuous bony tube which contains and protects the spinal cord. The hole in each vertebra through which the cord passes is called the *spinal canal*; the two holes at each level which permit spinal nerves to exit are called *intervertebral foramen*.

How Back Pain Is Generated

Some generalizations may be made about the origin of pain associated with the spinal column. For the sake of simplicity, it is best to outline and classify all the tissues from which pain can arise.

It is believed that some of the ligamentous tissue that holds vertebrae together is pain-sensitive. The ligamentum flavum and the interspinous ligaments are believed to be insensitive to pain, or at least minimally involved in the perception of pain.

The synovial lining and the articular capsule of the facet joints are richly supplied by sensory receptors or nerve endings. These joints are highly pain-sensitive.

Muscle spasm, which often accompanies spinal (joint) dysfunction and/or disease, can in itself elicit pain.

So it is that the pain from a back injury can result from a multitude of factors, including joint and ligamentous irritation and the sustained spasm of the muscle. Such multiple factors can be seen to contribute to the production of pain at each vertebral level. Other pain-sensitive tissues include nerves and blood vessels. In normal circumstances, however, this receptor system of nerve terminals located in and around the spine remains virtually inactive until irritated mechanically or chemically.

Testing for Low Back Disease

Patient's History

In back pain, as with the majority of medical disorders, the most important part of the examination is taking the patient's history: a description of *chief complaint*, which in this case is pain in the back, and its relation to *present illness*. Essential are the questions where, when, how, how much. Where is the pain? In the low back or in the buttocks? Does it go down one or both legs? Does the pain radiate up into the shoulders and neck? How did the pain start? Did it come gradually? Did it follow an injury or specific trauma? If so, when did that happen? What is the trend? Is the pain getting worse or better? Is it steady or intermittent?

The relationship to movement is very important. Does the pain increase with movement and decrease with rest (as in a mechanical back disorder) or — a most important sign — is there a great deal of night pain? The latter situation is usually associated with serious disease disorder.

Next is the question of *past history*. Have you ever had back pain before? If you did, what was the diagnosis? the treatment? How long did both pain and treatment last? *Occupational history* is important. What type of work do you do? What about other activities? How does the pain affect your home life, your sports or leisure activities, your sex life?

Family history is sometimes also important, especially when arthritis in the back is being considered. And finally: Are you in good health generally or are there other complaints in other organ systems? Are you taking other medications or treatments?

The physical examination should be done with the patient wearing only shorts or underpants and the practitioner looking not only at the low back region but also at the hips, the full back, and the legs. We encounter a surprising number of people who don't expect to have to undress for a back examination — having had such examinations previously while fully clothed. This is a shocking but telling revelation.

It's important for us to watch how people walk, to look at the curves in the low back and at the posture, and then to check the range of movement — the ability to extend the back backward, forward toward the toes — and feel the muscles on each side of the spine for muscle spasm and tenderness. Examination next entails a careful assessment of the pressure on nerve roots, which includes tests of muscle strength in hips, knees, ankles, and toes. Then come pin prick and other tests of sensory changes such as numbness or tingling in the lower extremities. Absent or diminished reflexes at the knee and ankle are sought. Finally, a test of straight-leg raising is done, where the patient lies on the back with body and legs straight out while the examiner raises each leg to a 90° angle (or as close to it as possible).

The physical examination will then expand to include other organs and other areas of the body. For most people, at this point, there are minimal findings. If disease has been ruled out, the patient will usually be treated with rest and painkillers, and perhaps some form of heat.

Low Back X-Rays

Other tests are usually indicated if a more serious disorder is suspected, if the pain is very intense, or if after initial treatment the pain has not settled down. The first of these tests is the low back X-ray — a very easy procedure that carries minimal radiation risk. X-rays are helpful in diagnosing fractures and *spondylolisthesis*, as we'll see, but simple X-rays rarely give useful information about the spine. The problem is that the spine often has minor abnormalities to which a pain source may be attributed. Often low back X-rays actually confuse the situation, producing erroneous diagnoses.

CATscan, MRI, Myelogram, and Other Tests

If pressure on a nerve root is indicated by examination, there are three other important tests (out of many available) that help to define this problem: CATscan, MRI, and Myelogram.

Computerized Axial Tomography (CATscan)
In a CATscan, multiple X-rays are taken and assimilated by a computer, giving a detailed, three-dimensional view of the low back. CATscan is an excellent means of assessing disease in the low back — from fractures to tumors and even soft-tissue injuries like herniated disc.

CATscan is noninvasive and carries very little risk for the patient. It is highly specific in localizing surgical lesions in the low back.

Magnetic Resonance Imagery (MRI)

MRI is a technique in which large magnets are used to create a magnetic field in the body, causing changes in the cells that are interpreted by way of color changes in the tissues to identify disease. This is also a noninvasive technique, but it has certain limitations.

Myelogram

Myelogram (*myelo* = spinal cord; *gram* = picture) is an invasive technique. A needle is placed between two vertebrae into the spinal canal, and radio opaque medium (a type of dye) is injected as the patient's body is tilted. The injection indicates whether there is nerve root pressure in a specific area. As with any invasive procedure, there are some risks of infection, along with the possibility of making the patient quite miserable for a few days with a headache or with discomfort in the low back.

Other Tests

Both blood tests and bone scans are helpful in determining when inflammatory disease is present in the low back. Bone scans use a medium that is labeled with radioactive isotopes and placed into a vein, where it is selectively attracted toward active inflammatory or growing bony tissue.

When Back Pain Is Caused by Disease

As we stated earlier, disease is the cause of back pain in a small minority of cases. The following are descriptions of these specific diseases that affect the back.*

Herniated Disc

Before we define herniated disc, let's first take a closer look at an *intervertebral disc*. Each flat surface of a vertebra is covered with articular cartilage. Between each pair of vertebrae is the disc, its fluid-like interior core covered by criss-crossing fibers in layers that are

---

* See chapter 10 for case histories.

much like those of an onion. The outermost layers of the disc blend with intervertebral ligaments to join the vertebrae together. The normal, healthy disc acts as a shock absorber.

Originally the disc was thought to be a static structure, but we now know that the disc imbibes fluid at night and, because of the activity and weight of our bodies, exudes it through the day. This process could be compared to squeezing water out of a sponge. For this reason, the height of each disc lessens as the day goes on, causing our overall height to decrease.

Herniated disc is a rupture of the outer layer of fibers, which allows the inner gelatinous disc material to exude (see figure 2.5). The condition was first described in an operation in 1934. Upon removal of the disc fragment that was putting pressure on a nerve, the patient lost the "sciatic" pain and recovery was quick and complete. Although this discovery received scant attention initially, its significance would eventually reach inappropriate levels.

FIG. 2.5 HERNIATED DISC

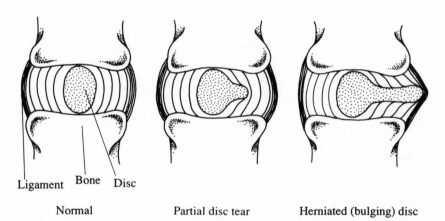

Ligament   Bone   Disc

Normal   Partial disc tear   Herniated (bulging) disc

The manifestations of herniated disc are many and varied. They are related to the different phases of the disease process in the disc itself and to the secondary changes occurring in the surrounding tissues. Invariably the patient seeks professional aid because of pain in the low back, with or without pain in one or both legs. The nature of the pain is governed by pressure on the components of the nerve roots, if they are involved, and by the stimulation or irritation of the surrounding ligaments (see figure 2.6).

When the gelatinous material of a disc herniates, the character and the intensity of the symptoms depend not only upon the size and direction of the herniation but upon the shape and size of the spinal canal.

Herniated disc occurs in 0.1 to 0.5 percent of males between the ages of 24 and 64 — most commonly around age 30. It is even less common in women. A patient may have experienced previous low back pain, but not necessarily. The most common occurrence is when a young, healthy disc herniates under high pressure. The individual knows at once that something is wrong, even though there may be no low back pain *at the time* of the herniation; rather there is a numbness or weakness in one or both legs. In extreme cases, the patient also loses bladder and bowel control.

In testing for herniated disc, the function of the nerve roots to the lower leg must be checked. Symptoms of nerve root pressure or irritation are pain or numbness in one or both legs, loss of reflexes, and/or weakness of muscles in the legs as well as a limitation of straight-leg elevation from the horizontal position.

FIG. 2.6 **DISC HERNIATION**

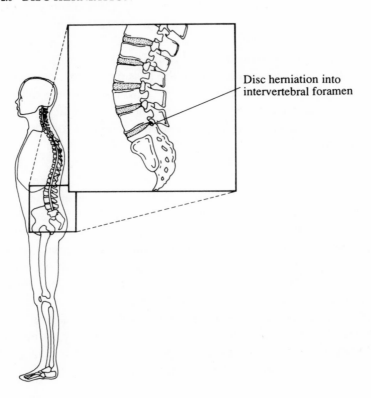

Disc herniation into intervertebral foramen

Most herniated discs will retract or shrivel up in time (three to nine months), causing a natural relief of pressure and pain. In severe or progressive cases, operative treatment may be indicated. The level of the lesion is ascertained by a myelogram, CATscan, or other test, and then the disc may be chemically dissolved by an enzyme or surgically removed by a discotomy. In some cases, the nerve root is so pressured by disc and surrounding bone that a small piece of bone is removed in the connecting arch. This procedure is called a *laminectomy*.

Ankylosing Spondylitis

This condition, also called Marie Strumpell disease, is a form of inflammatory arthritis. The disease is often familial, is predominant in males at a five-to-one ratio to females, and affects up to 4 percent of all those who suffer with back pain.

The onset is usually between ages 25 and 35 and is manifest in low back discomfort characterized by stiffness of one or both buttocks at the base of the spine. This stiffness is more apparent after an individual has remained in the same position for a prolonged period and is particularly apparent upon awakening in the morning.

In its early stages, ankylosing spondylitis is rather insidious and tends to be episodic, with its onset usually only vaguely recalled by the patient during consultation. With the passing of time, however, the episodes of discomfort become more and more severe and may awaken the patient from a sound sleep during the night. Eventually, these episodes are superseded by increased aching and stiffness, which are aggravated by inactivity.

Over a period of years, the increasingly severe episodes of pain are associated with increasing rigidity of the spine. As the disease proceeds, it causes fusion of the vertebrae and can eventually also cause bony fusion of the ligaments, producing the rigid, solid spine that we call "bamboo spine." Individuals with this condition have little spinal movement and walk like robots. Without corrective treatment, ankylosing spondylitis can also cause locking or fusion of the rib cage, resulting in a barrel chest with little flexibility and in impairment of breathing. Fatigue is another effect of the disease.

The primary approach to treating patients with this active arthritic condition is to keep them moving about as much as possible. Anti-inflammatory medication helps one aspect of the problem, but patients get into serious difficulties if they decide to simply "pack it in" and rest.

Spondylolisthesis (Unstable Spine)

S pondylolisthesis is a condition of forward sliding of the body of one vertebra on the vertebra below it. The term is derived from the Greek word *olisthesis*, which means a slipping or falling. It is the most common cause of instability or excessive movement in the spine (see figure 2.7).

FIG. 2.7 **SPONDYLOLITHESIS**

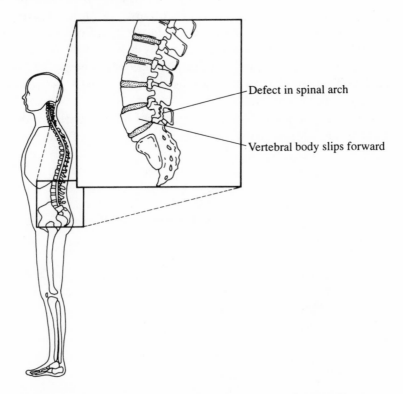

Defect in spinal arch

Vertebral body slips forward

Spondylolisthesis may occur anywhere along the spinal column, but most commonly occurs at the last lumbar vertebra, L5. It results from a defect of the spinal arch. When a defect in the spinal arch exists alone with no slippage, it is called a *spondylolysis*; this usually does not cause pain.

Pain in the low back attributable to spondylolisthesis undoubtedly results from the strain imposed on the holding elements (the ligaments and the intervertebral joints).

Surgical intervention is indicated for severe slippage and also indicated if the slippage causes pressure on a nerve root (*sciatica*). In this operation, two vertebrae are fused or joined together, with bone taken from the patient's hip joint. It is called *vertebral fusion*.

Trauma to Low Back

The most common cause of trauma to the spine is a *compression fracture* of the vertebral body (see figure 2.8). A compressive force to the bone causes it to collapse inward, usually in a wedgelike manner, causing severe pain for many weeks. Treatment is usually by bed rest, and occasionally a body cast is used if the damage is extensive or at multiple vertebral levels. In younger people, fracture as such is a rare occurrence, usually the result of a car accident or a bad fall.

About 25 percent of older women and 12 percent of older men suffer from *osteoporosis*, or severe deterioration of the bones. Of

FIG. 2.8 VERTEBRAL FRACTURE

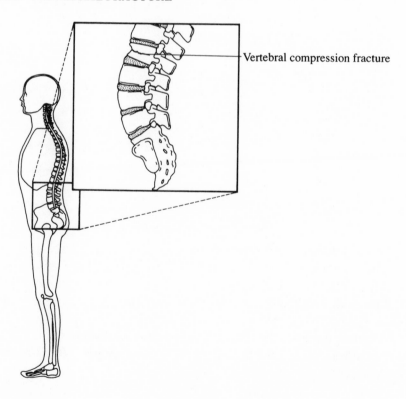

Vertebral compression fracture

approximately six million spontaneous fractures that occur in North America in a year, postmenopausal women sustain about five million. These spontaneous fractures are often the first sign of the disease, although the first symptom in postmenopausal women is pain in the low back area, which becomes progressively worse.

Osteoporosis, which represents a decrease in the total bone mass in the body without actual change in chemical composition of the bones (the ratio of calcium to protein remains normal), also causes loss of height at a rate of about 1.5 inches per decade after menopause has begun. In approximately 26 percent of women over 60, resultant vertebral deformities cause "dowager's hump."

Metastatic (Spreading) Disease

We are referring here to primary disease elsewhere in the body which produces back pain. With metastatic cancer, for example, the primary disease in women is most commonly located in the

FIG. 2.9 INTERNAL DISEASE MANIFEST IN THE SPINE

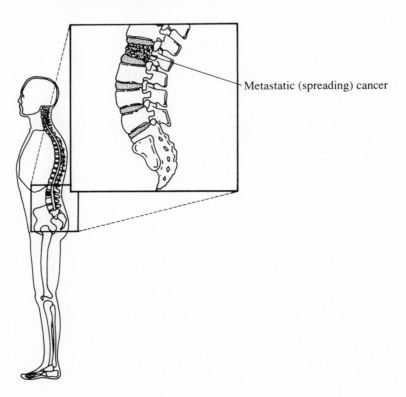

Metastatic (spreading) cancer

reproductive organs or the breast; in men, the location is most frequently in the colon or the prostate. Spinal pain in these cases is thus a secondary phenomenon and requires accurate diagnosis and treatment of the underlying causative disease. Internal disease manifest in the spine is illustrated in figure 2.9.

Degenerative Disc Disease

The degenerative process preceding disc disease is the object of wide discussion. Its origin and presence do not enjoy conformity of interpretation. Much is known about disc anatomy and chemistry, but it is the mechanical function that is important in interpreting disc breakdown and deviation from the norm.

The intervertebral disc can be described as a hydraulic system composed of a fibro-elastic cylinder filled with a colloidal gel. As mentioned earlier, the discs comprise one-quarter of the supporting spine structure of the human body. In youth, the discs are springy and under high positive pressure, forcing the vertebrae far apart. With age, however, the discs lose fluid content, intactness, and elasticity. The net effect is a loosening of the annular ligaments and a resulting shimmy. On X-ray, the condition may have the appearance of arthritis (and is sometimes called that), with small protuberances called *osteophytes* projecting from the edge of the vertebrae (see figure 2.10). It is not a true arthritis, however, but simply the result of wear and tear.

At about 40, many people begin to show degenerative disc disease on X-ray. At 60, everyone shows evidence of it. Many people simply put up with the pain that degenerative disc disease can cause. Although degenerative disc disease is a structural problem it behaves with a functional impact, and as such it can be alleviated or at least reduced.

It should be noted here, however, that degenerative disc disease does not necessarily produce pain. Nor can the appearance of the spine in X-ray be taken as an indicator of the presence of pain. Toronto orthopedic surgeon Ian Macnab proved this point in a study conducted at the Workmen's Compensation Hospital, where the backs of a number of heavy laborers were X-rayed. The study revealed that some individuals with dreadful-looking back X-rays reported experiencing no pain at all; conversely, patients with back problems often had quite normal-looking X-rays.

Yet the most common diagnosis we hear from patients themselves is "I have degenerating discs," and, further, "there's nothing to be done

FIG. 2.10   **DEGENERATIVE DISC DISEASE**

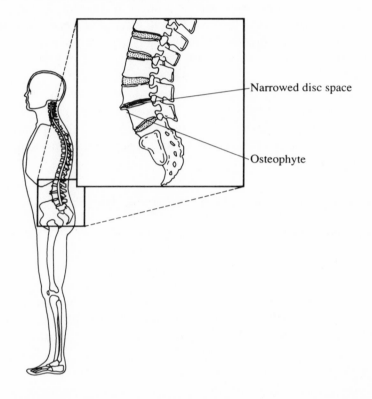

Narrowed disc space

Osteophyte

about it; I have to live with it." This elevation of a normal aging phenomenon to disease status can be very distressing and disabling to a patient.

In a similar frame of reference, we could tell an aging patient with graying or white hair that he or she has "degenerating scalp" and let that be interpreted as it might! Although back pain can be associated with degenerating discs, far too often it is cited as the cause of the problem.

Incidence of Disease

In 1975, Dr. A. Magora reported on a study he had undertaken involving 429 patients with low back pain. Dr. Magora is a neurosurgeon, and so he sees very difficult back cases. This is a skewed sample, then, in which all the cases reported may be regarded as extreme and unresponsive to normal conservative treatment approaches — the true "basket cases."

The results showed that after careful examination of these 429 patients with serious low back pain, a total of 72 percent showed *no evidence of neurological deficits or neurological problems*. Sixty-six percent had *no orthopedic findings at all*. Only 3 percent had evidence of herniated discs and/or pinched nerves, and just over 10 percent had hip findings.

This was amazing. Even in such a skewed sample as this, 66 percent of 429 patients had back pain *but no clinical findings*. They had a symptom, but they had *no specific disease*. Most of these people could not be given a diagnosis relating to any of the structural abnormalities we have just discussed.

Back Pain without Disease: The Overwhelming Majority

B eing health professionals, we know that patients have certain expectations. If they are suffering from back pain, they want to know why. The fact of the matter is that in only *5 to 10 percent* of the patients we see can we identify a specific disease as the cause of their pain. An overwhelming *90 percent* of individuals with back pain have no structural abnormalities/disease, even though most people we see have initially made the assumption that they do. *What is causing their pain?*

Back Pain: A Symptom of What?

A fter cool reflection on the current state of affairs, we can un- equivocally state that most back pain cannot, in good scientific terms, be attributed to any specific disease process that can be treated by medical or surgical means. But patients and doctors alike, accustomed to the successes of the medical disease model, expect a diagnosis. "I don't know for sure what's wrong" does not raise one's professional esteem or a patient's confidence.

When examination results are minimal, the usual course is to order an X-ray of the spine. Where an X-ray shows no low back findings, the patient's back pain has traditionally been called something: "lumbar sprain" or "back strain" or "muscle spasm." For individuals over 40 it has been traditionally labeled as degenerative and "something you'll have to live with."

Specific diseases such as herniated disc or ankylosing spondylitis have specific findings or criteria on which all practitioners would agree with the diagnosis. But lumbar sprain or degenerative disc disease are more like the "flu." Those names can mean virtually anything you want them to. These terms for back pain seem to satisfy both practitioner and patient that a specific disease entity is present. Then the symptom, *back pain*, instead of the underlying disease, becomes the objective of treatment. All efforts are now made to modulate or reduce pain. All success is measured by the degree of pain reduction and the length of time in which pain disappears.

Fortunately, Mother Nature is on our side. Statistics indicate that

45 percent of back pain disappears in one week,
80 percent of back pain disappears in 4 weeks, and
90 percent of back pain disappears in 8 weeks

regardless of the type of treatment. A cynic might add that the last treatment undertaken usually gets the credit for the cure.

Is this a desperate situation? Is there a better approach to this "hidden epidemic"?

What we want to stress in the next two chapters — and throughout this book — is this: Where back pain is not produced by a specific disease with specific treatment to deal with the *cause*, the problem is usually one of a *functional disorder. The vast majority of patients who suffer from back pain can learn self-help and self-management of their problems — can learn to be the best they can be — with professional guidance.*

One of the cornerstones of our approach to this whole subject is that of back *function versus dysfunction* . . . how each individual *uses* and at times *misuses* the back. Taking this functional approach, we shall show you how to alleviate back pain *as much as is possible for you.* And if you have yet to suffer from back pain, humankind's most persistent complaint, you will learn how to *prevent or minimize* its occurrence.

Nor does this approach of management of back pain stop when the pain disappears. Rather, it is the beginning of a process of care and maintenance for optimal back health for a lifetime. This approach creates a climate that also reduces the chances of severe disability developing in that unfortunate 10 percent of sufferers whose back pain does not go away spontaneously.

3

Normal Function of the Low Back

In looking at normal back function, we're going to describe and explain what the back has been designed to do. We'll explain how the back works, when it is working properly, and when it is *used* properly. Let's first consider the general concept of function.

Function: What It Means

If you begin to notice some impairment of vision — you may have started to have difficulty reading the fine print in the phone book, for example — you'll have the *function* of your eyes tested. You'll start by having a functional rather than a disease examination. (In a minority of cases, disease *will* be present; regardless, the problem is one of function, and that must be examined initially.)

If your eyes are found not to be working properly, glasses will more than likely be prescribed to correct the problem.

The same applies should you begin to notice hearing loss or impairment. The doctor will first test the function of your ears and if a disorder is found, will probably prescribe a hearing aid to correct the problem. Again, not usually a question of disease, but rather of dysfunction.

If you've led a sedentary life-style for a time and one day decide to go out jogging, you're going to come back wheezing, coughing, and winded. The next day you'll notice stiffness and may feel tired. Will you go to the doctor about it? No. You'll recognize the symptoms of dysfunction. You're out of shape, but you're not ill. And you realize that if you increase this new daily exercise at a sensible rate, you'll gradually decrease your dysfunction. Stated another way, you'll *improve the function* of your limbs, heart, and lungs.

In talking about the back, we'll make the same point: simply because a back is weak or painful or not working properly, that does not mean disease is present. As we've seen, disease accounts for no more than 5-10 percent of back problems. What is present in most cases is *mechanical low back dysfunction*, which can cause pain just as unaccustomed exercise can cause pain in the unfit runner.

Before we look at mechanical low back dysfunction, however, let's be absolutely clear about normal function of the low back.

Normal Back Function

As pictured in figure 3.1. The back has two basic functions: first, to provide strong, stable foundation for weight-bearing because the spine is the major load-transmitting structure of the human body; and second, to permit flexibility in movement, without which we would move and walk like robots.

FIG. 3.1 **TWO FUNCTIONAL MODES OF THE SPINE**

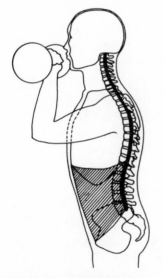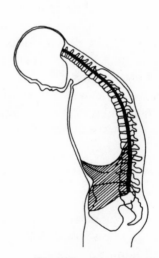

Stability, for weight-bearing   Flexibility, for movement

A third, peripheral, function of the spinal column is as a bony framework to protect the vital spinal cord, which acts as the brain's message-carrier to limbs and organs. The spine must be able to sustain heavy loads without excessive deformation or movement in order to ensure that the spinal cord is completely protected from injury.

The Mechanics of Movement

How surprising that the two main functions of the back should apparently be incompatible. On one level, the back permits flexibility of movement. But for stability and weight-bearing, a strong foundation with no movement — as with a house — is needed.

For a clear understanding of how the body moves, let's first look at the components involved: the bony *skeleton*, which supports the body; ligaments, which attach bones to form joints; and the *muscles*, which provide the moving force.

The skeleton is the main supporting structure of the body. It is composed of rigid bones that, by their arrangement, contribute to body shape and stability. The bones are of various sizes, shapes, and densities — each designed to carry out its particular function. The long bones of the legs, for example, are large and strong for weight-bearing, whereas the bones of the skull and face are light so that the head can be supported with ease. The chainlike arrangement of the spine allows for great flexibility in motion and is also the center for muscular attachment.

Ligaments are the strong cords that join bones together, and a joint is the place where two bones meet. Usually, though not always, the structure of a joint allows motion of one or both of these bones.

Skeletal muscles move the skeleton and are attached to bones by strong, fibrous cords called tendons. Skeletal muscles are capable of rapid, powerful contraction or of prolonged periods of *partial* contraction (maintaining posture). The muscles of the back cross the bony joints and either stabilize them or create movement.

The Spinal Column: Our Central Support System

The spinal column, itself a support mechanism, likewise depends on bony supports, ligamentous supports, and muscular supports.

A healthy low back will show the characteristics of normal or balanced joint movement in the bones; ligamentous support that contributes to normal posture; and balanced, strong, and flexible muscles.

Bony Supports
The Joint   Where two bones come together to form a joint, the function is usually to permit movement in the bony skeleton. The ends of the bones that meet in a joint are covered by *cartilage* — a soft,

spongy "bone" substance that works as a shock absorber. Figure 3.2 illustrates an elbow joint.

FIG. 3.2 ELBOW JOINT (EXAMPLE OF A JOINT)

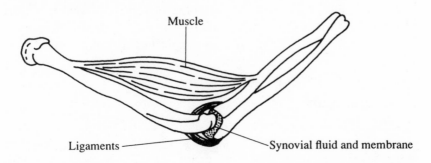

In the low back, each vertebra has three joints: two facet joints and one disc joint. As we saw in the previous chapter, the vertebra consists of the strong, square anterior "body" with a semicircular ring at the back to which the two facet joints are attached. These facet joints are similar to the "generic" joint just described, consisting of bone and cartilage joined by ligaments.

The disc joint, however, is a modified type of joint. The bones are joined by ligaments, but the cartilage has effectively been replaced by the gelatinous disc (described in the previous chapter). The basic function of the disc joint is weight-bearing rather than movement.

The basic unit of function in the low back is thus two adjacent vertebrae, the three joints of each vertebra, the ligaments that link the joints, and the muscles that support them. These components are illustrated in figure 3.3.

FIG. 3.3 TWO FACET JOINTS AND ONE DISC JOINT LINK AT EACH SPINAL LEVEL

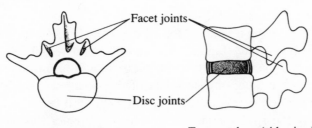

Stability/Weight-Bearing Mode   In healthy function, the main force of bearing weight must be taken by the strong, anterior disc joints of the vertebrae. The posterior facet joints, designed for movement, simply do not bear weight well.

As well, the position of the vertebrae is very important to ensure that the functional unit works safely. Figure 3.4 shows the normal vertebral and disc position, with no weight-bearing taking place; and, for comparison, the neutral or normal position of the vertebrae functioning to support weight correctly.

FIG. 3.4   **DISC JOINT**

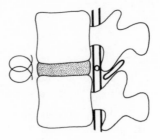

A. Not bearing weight

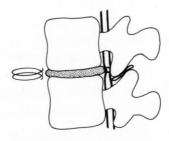

B. Bearing weight (compression of disc)

If, however, weight-bearing forces go through the facet joints as a result of poor posture (figure 3.5), not only is there the risk of these joints becoming jammed or injured, but there will be a tilting or shearing force on the anterior disc joints of the vertebrae. Further, if the forces are exerted in this way, the spinal canal will become narrowed, thus placing the spinal cord and its nerves at greater risk. (Posture is discussed in more detail in the following chapter.)

FIG. 3.5 POOR POSTURE: WEIGHT-BEARING FORCES GOING THROUGH FACET JOINTS

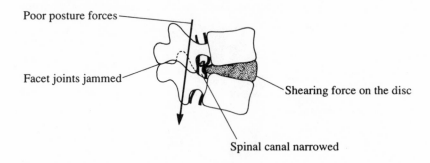

Poor posture forces

Facet joints jammed

Shearing force on the disc

Spinal canal narrowed

Flexibility/Movement Mode Most movement in the low back occurs at the facet joints, which are similar in appearance to dishes placed on end and sliding one on another. In the low back, movement is mainly a function of one dishlike joint sliding parallel to another. Actions that cause twisting in the low back can cause jamming of these facet joints because they are not being used within their correct range of movement. Figure 3.6 illustrates flexion and backward extension in the flexibility mode.

FIG. 3.6 FLEXIBILITY MODE

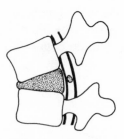 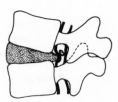

A. Flexion of spine   B. Backward extension of spine

The Spinal Column The spinal column is made up of a multiple of functional units stacked one on top of the other (figure 3.7). The five lumbar vertebrae create six functional units, which we like to call the *working unit*. The working unit has the two functions of stability and movement, as well as the protective function for the spinal cord and nerves. Again, note the importance of good posture.

FIG. 3.7 WORKING UNIT FORMING THE SPINAL COLUMN

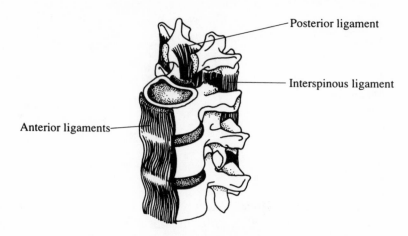

(shows 3 of the 5 lumbar vertebrae ligaments)

Pelvic Ring: The Vital Connector   As the human body's major weight-transmitting structure, the spine cannot float in isolation. Rather, it must be connected through the legs and feet to the ground. The vital connector that performs this function is called the *pelvic ring*.

The pelvic ring consists of three bones: the *sacrum* and two *innominate* (hip) bones, the latter connected to the *femurs* (thigh bones). Together, these three bones form five joints: two *sacroiliac joints* at the base of the spine; two *hip joints* where the hip bones join the legs; and the *symphysis pubis*, where the two hip bones join in the front. Figure 3.8 provides a frontal and side view, showing both the link and the "couple" at this area.

FIG. 3.8 THE PELVIC RING

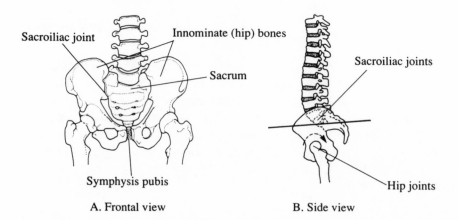

Normal Function of the Pelvic Ring   During normal standing or sitting, the ligaments of the sacroiliac joints and the pelvic ring are loose. When weight-bearing occurs, the pressure exerted down through the spinal column would force the sacrum downward, were it not for the diagonally placed sacroiliac ligaments that now tighten up.

This tightening causes the pelvic ring to go from its neutral or loose position into a tight, coiled position, allowing greater stability. Through the pelvic ring, weight is transmitted down through the legs to the ground. A key characteristic of the pelvic ring is its strong ligamentous support, which is particularly important during weight-bearing. If this support is breached, it will create significant dysfunction in the low spine, both in walking and in weight-bearing.

A second key feature of the pelvic ring is that its position of tilt determines the quality of the curves in the spinal column above it. If the pelvic ring is in a relatively safe, balanced position, the curves in the spinal column will be normally balanced and the posture safe. If the pelvic ring is excessively tilted one way or the other, however, the spine will have poor posture, and be dysfunctional and susceptible to injury. (The pelvic ring is discussed in further detail in chapter 6.)

Ligamentous Supports

As seen in figure 3.9 the spine is supported by *anterior (front) ligaments*, *posterior (behind) ligaments*, and *interspinous (between the spines of the vertebrae) ligaments*. Pelvic ligaments join the spine to the pelvis and link the three pelvic bones to form the pelvic ring. Their function is to permit a healthy range of movement in the low spine. Excessive movement of the spine, however, will put these ligaments under unnecessary dysfunctional stress and strain.

FIG. 3.9 LIGAMENTS SUPPORTING THE SPINE

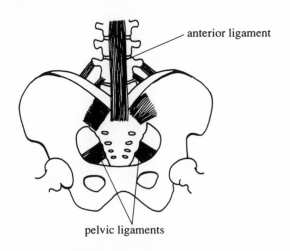

anterior ligament

pelvic ligaments

Muscular Supports

Even with the best bony and ligamentous supports, the spine cannot remain erect and fight the force of gravity on its own. Bones and ligaments, which are static elements, must be maintained in their upright position by dynamic muscular support.

There are hundreds of separate muscles in the low back, and their classification is highly complex. For the sake of simplicity, we'll divide the primary trunk or low back muscles into four main groups: back muscles, stomach muscles, sling muscles, and lateral muscles.

Back muscles (figure 3.10) are situated in two columns on either side of the central spinal column, supporting the spine from the back. They can be easily felt with the hands.

Stomach muscles (figure 3.11) extend from the symphysis pubis and pelvic ring, giving frontal or anterior support to the spine. Very thin muscles, they are extremely important because they operate at a distance from the spine and so have a leverage effect.

FIG. 3.10 BACK MUSCLES   **FIG. 3.11 STOMACH MUSCLES**

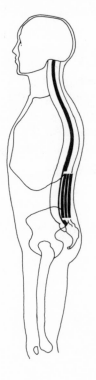
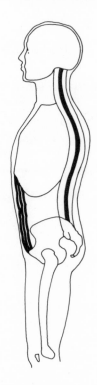

Sling muscles or hip flexors (figure 3.12) link the transverse processes of the spine on the inside, cross the pelvic ring, and attach to the thigh bones just below the hip. They are crucial in maintaining upright posture.

Lateral (side) muscles (figure 3.13) are located between the rib cage and the pelvic ring. They flow over the pelvic ring in and around the hip area and down into the leg.

FIG. 3.12 SLING MUSCLES   **FIG. 3.13 LATERAL (SIDE) MUSCLES**

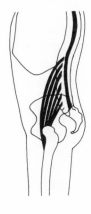

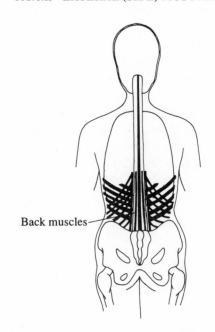

Back muscles

These four groups comprise the primary trunk or low back muscles. Also important for support are two types of secondary supporting muscles: the *quadriceps* (thigh muscles), which extend down the front of the thighs to the kneecaps; and the *hamstrings*, which attach to the pelvic ring and go down the backs of the thighs to attach behind the knees. The quadriceps and hamstrings contribute to the tilt or balance of the pelvic ring.

Muscular Supports and Spinal Function   Muscles function mainly by contracting. Although muscle contraction creates movement of the low back, excessive contraction can take movement *out of* the low back. A simple illustration of this action can be seen in this *wrist* demonstration:

Slowly contract and relax the muscles that support your wrist (they're called *flexors* and *extensors*). The wrist will move freely. Now, firmly contract those muscles, as in a punching position. The wrist has become stable. All movement and flexibility have gone out of the wrist.

In just the same way, the muscles that support the spine can relax and contract to create movement and flexibility, *or* they can all solidly contract together to create a solid, inflexible, and robotlike weight-bearing or stable mode.

Stomach Support Mechanism   When the trunk muscles contract strongly, they compress the contents of the abdominal area — stomach, intestines, and fat. This action creates a stomach support mechanism (figure 3.14) that helps to bear weight and distribute it more evenly throughout the spine.

The stomach support function can be compared to that of a water-bed, where water is enclosed within a large, flat container and will bear weight so long as that "integrity of containment" is maintained. The contraction of the trunk muscles creates a similar mechanism to bear weight and support the spine in the weight-bearing mode.

FIG. 3.14 STOMACH SUPPORT MECHANISM

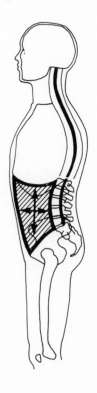

Muscles and Posture   It is, finally, our muscles that create the posture or position of the spine so crucial to maintaining functional spinal health. The key to maintaining good posture is correct position of the pelvic ring — a *balanced* position — so that the spinal column above the pelvic ring is not excessively curved backward or forward (figures 3.15, 3.16).

FIG. 3.15 GOOD POSTURE   **FIG. 3.16 POOR POSTURE**

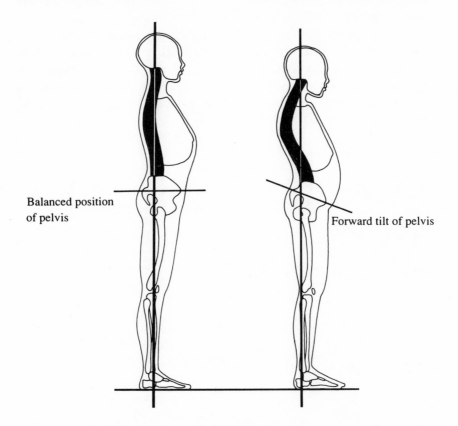

Balanced position
of pelvis

Forward tilt of pelvis

So it is that the muscles, dynamic in function, create normal posture, which is balanced, or permit abnormal posture, which can cause dysfunctional loads to be placed on the bones and ligaments.

Summary

In summing up, let us repeat that proper and healthy function of the back means the ability to have *full flexibility and movement*, within the structural limitations of the joint: forward, backward, and sideways. It also means the ability or strength to contract the trunk muscles *to eliminate movement* in the stable or weight-bearing mode. As well, healthy function means *good posture* — healthy curves in the low back to transmit normal forces properly through the spine.

To understand the mechanics by which the spine can accommodate these seemingly incompatible functions of stability and mobility, it is necessary to understand that all three functional elements of the low back — the static bones and ligaments and the dynamic muscles — must interact harmoniously to form an efficient functioning unit.

A *pain-free back* may be a functioning back or it may be a back that is dysfunctioning to a minor degree which, if allowed to continue, may become severe enough to produce low back pain. In the next chapter, we shall look at dysfunction of the low back and spine.

4

Dysfunction of the Low Back and Spine

As we have seen, complex as it is the spine has been beautifully engineered and designed for those two seemingly incompatible functions: creating stability and creating movement.

The Biomechanical Approach

Organic disease is the cause of low back pain in fewer than 10 percent of cases. Much more common are *biomechanical* (bio = living/mechanical) abnormalities, which produce overloading of the spinal structures. The bones, ligaments, and muscles that comprise these structures can be stressed in various ways because of forces continually acting on the spine.

For example, there are compressive forces that push bones and discs together; this happens when we lift a weight. There are tension or tensile forces that act on ligaments and muscles, as happens when we bend forward in an extreme position. And there are shearing or twisting forces that can act gradually over a long period of time (from being subjected to abnormal postures in the workplace, for example) or can have a sudden effect (a fall on a football field, down a ski slope, or on an icy parking lot).

Harmony of muscle function is necessary for maintaining normal spinal and postural function. Although there is little doubt that injury or overuse may be the initial culprit responsible for altering joint mechanics, the more subtle or insidious stresses usually associated with life-style are seldom recognized as the precipitating factors of musculoskeletal-related pain syndromes.

Dysfunction (abnormal function) usually begins with a deterioration in muscle harmony and may go unnoticed for years or even decades. As the muscle physiology changes in terms of length or tone, so does its function. And because muscles move bones, the result is a change in the axis of motion around which all joints must move. This alteration in the axis of motion has a detrimental effect on some of the structural elements in and around the joints.

Characteristics of the Dysfunctional Back

A dysfunctional back may or may not produce pain. Abnormal motion will be present, but there will be no obvious structural lesion at first; that is, no disease element.

Patients whose backs are dysfunctional cannot use their spine correctly, and the resulting postural stress affects the functional interaction between muscles and joints. Muscle spasm and joint stiffness alter the mechanics at the affected segments. This process may continue for months or even years until such time as early pathological changes occur.

The dysfunctional phase involves muscles and joints primarily; if pain is present, it arises from facet joints that are improperly used or overloaded and/or from muscle overload. As the process continues, soft tissue is compromised, and increased abnormal movement (instability or hypermobility) is added to the pre-existing dysfunction.

The final phase is visible on X-ray. Gross pathological changes result in wear and tear of the cartilage tissue covering the facet joints, and an increased surface area of the vertebral body is seen as bony projections (osteophytes). Further trauma will likely again lead to instability, which over a period of years may become more severe.

Dysfunction of the Spine: The Causes

There are four primary causes of dysfunction of the spine: (1) degenerative disc disease; (2) abnormal postures; (3) muscle dysfunction or reaction to injury; and (4) segmental changes to joints. Each of these will be discussed in turn.

Degenerative Disc Disease

Degenerative disc disease (figure 4.1), as mentioned in the preceding chapter, is a normal aging process that all individuals go through. With some people, however, the spine ages faster than with others. X-rays show evidence of degenerative disc disease in most people by about age 40, and in all people by age 60. It is caused primarily by loss of fluid — or aging — in the discs. As a result, the discs become less resilient, permitting two vertebrae to move closer together. We consider the term to be a misnomer; degenerative disc disease is an *aging process*, not unlike that of hair turning gray.

FIG. 4.1 DEGENERATIVE DISC DISEASE

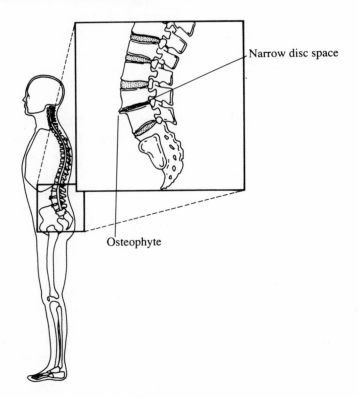

Narrow disc space

Osteophyte

Dysfunctions Caused by Degenerative Disc Disease

In degenerative disc disease, the ligaments that join the bodies of the vertebrae become looser, permitting a shimmy between the bones. The facet joints, which permit movement when functioning normally, jam closer together, decreasing flexibility. The intervertebral foramen, where the nerves of the spinal cord exit, become smaller, permitting a greater chance of pressure on a nerve or nerves — a condition called *spinal stenosis*. And now, because of the shimmy caused by loosened ligaments, the muscles are called upon to work harder. The extra work makes the muscles more tense, often with accompanying pain or stiffness.

This aging process may result in stiffness and in some degree of low back pain, or in greater susceptibility to more major problems, such as the stenosis noted above. It happens at different rates in different people, but we all go through it.

Abnormal Postures

In the physiological sense, posture means a certain orientation of the body in space (the act of standing) or of the components of the body in relation to one another. Although each of us has an individual posture, we all oppose the same force of gravity — a continuous battle that involves the mechanisms for maintaining balance or, if need be, restoring balance.

Our upright stance imposes an extreme mechanical disadvantage, so the body functions on the principle of taking the path of least resistance. In terms of posture, this means that once an individual has learned to adapt to a poor or slumped stance or sitting position, any attempts to use the relevant muscles correctly may feel awkward and may soon cause discomfort. As this abnormal pattern becomes habitual, the original muscles weaken and tend to atrophy from disuse. Abnormal patterns of this kind may result in muscle imbalance, and the deformity becomes progressively worse.

The Most Common Types of Poor Posture
The most common types of poor posture are: (1) an increase or decrease of the curve of the low back and (2) a slumping or slouching of the shoulders (outward curvature).

Figure 4.2 illustrates the most frequently seen defects, which are: (1) the *round-shouldered* back; (2) *the flat back*; (3) *the lordotic back*; and (4) *scoliosis* (lateral curvature of the spine).

Effects of Abnormal Postures
On *discs*, abnormal posture can create pressure, which causes undue wear and tear and may even result in a ruptured or herniated disc. On *ligaments*, the result can be strain and loosening. On *muscles*, abnormal posture can create a condition called *static loading*.

To illustrate static-muscle loading (figure 4.3), take two weights or heavy books that weigh about five pounds each. Hold one in each hand; put one arm down at your side, and stretch the other arm full-length sideways. The dangling arm can maintain its position for quite a long time. The outstretched arm, however, creates static-muscle

FIG. 4.2 FREQUENTLY SEEN POSTURE DEFECTS

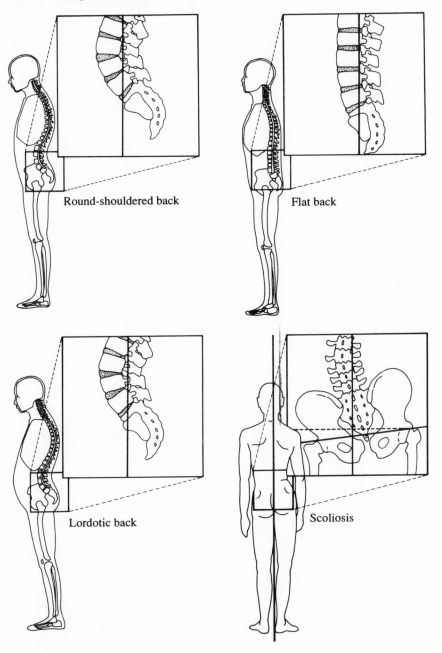

Round-shouldered back

Flat back

Lordotic back

Scoliosis

loading in the shoulder muscles and can remain in its position for only a few minutes without significant discomfort.

FIG. 4.3 **STATIC MUSCLE STRAIN (ILLUSTRATED ON SHOULDER MUSCLES)**

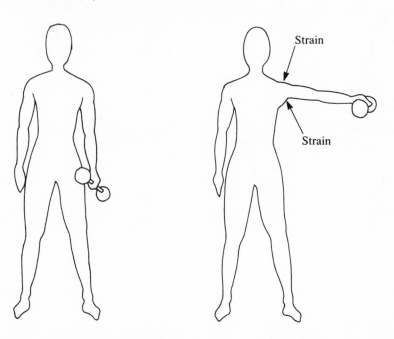

Maintaining this static-loaded posture with the arm outstretched causes the individual to expend an excess amount of energy unnecessarily. Bad posture has the same effect, which leads to fatigue by the end of the day. The secretary who leans over a desk day after day develops tight, sore muscles at the base of the neck and in the shoulders. With time the stronger muscles will take over and lead to a muscular imbalance surrounding the neck and shoulders. This imbalance then intrudes into everyday activities, as the secretary learns to move with the wrong group of muscles. The result is excessive wear and tear on the surrounding joints, leading usually to fatigue, irritability, and headaches, which are then attributed to tension. It is a situation that can arise in a multitude of occupations and activities. Unless individuals take adequate counter-measures, their body mechanics can be destroyed, resulting in permanent malformations.

Muscle Tone

In healthy individuals, muscles do not relax completely but maintain a slight degree of contraction, referred to as *muscle tone*. When muscles are not exercised regularly — as the result of disease, inactivity, or improper activity — they lose their tone and become long and flabby. Muscles that are long and flabby do not contract as powerfully as they should.

How Muscles become Dysfunctional

Abnormal forces as diverse as bad posture, injury, or stress create a shortened muscle that does not contract powerfully.

The following demonstration (illustrated in figure 4.4) shows that muscle health is a balanced muscle, neither too long nor too short, that can contract properly.

1) Position your right wrist (left wrist, if left-handed) as shown in A (the best balanced position) and grasp two fingers of your left hand. Squeeze as hard as possible.

2) Position your right wrist as shown in B (the short contracted muscle position). Now squeeze. Weaker, isn't it?

3) Position your right wrist as shown in C (the long, stretched muscle postion). Squeeze. Weaker, right?

FIG. 4.4 THE MUSCLE LENGTH-POWER CURVE

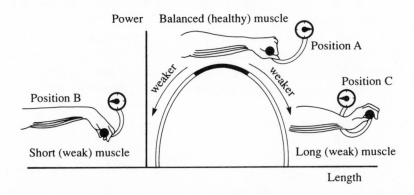

Injury produces painful muscle spasm and muscle shortening. Even after the pain disappears, the affected muscles remain short, weak, and more susceptible to future injury.

Stress for some people brings on low back pain or neck pain. This "uptight" feeling creates tight, tense muscles that are more susceptible to back injury.

With *aging*, our muscles tend to shorten — not because they have to, but because most people do not maintain active joint movements through daily stretching exercises.

Too much exercise or heavy manual work can cause tight, short muscles. This activity creates the "musclebound" condition of a short, contracted muscle that is a characteristic of weight lifters who do not warm up with stretching exercises.

In assessing low back dysfunction, it is important to look for muscle imbalance: muscles that are weak because they are too long or because they are too short.

Changes to Joints

A joint can become dysfunctional in two ways: it can become fixed, stiff, and immobile, meaning an overall loss of movement; or it can become unstable or hypermobile, with too much movement.

In the case of a loss of movement, the ligaments will usually be much tighter, with muscles losing their flexibility as well.

Where the joint has become unstable, the ligaments will in turn become loose and unstable, with the muscles becoming tense and sore in an attempt to compensate for and minimize the excessive movement.

Because the low back has many segments, fixation at one joint will mean compensatory changes producing hypermobility at adjacent joints.

The goal of spinal adjustive procedures, often referred to as spinal manipulation, is to correct dysfunction and the problems resulting from locked joints or restricted joint movement. A spinal joint that has reduced mobility is said to be in a state of fixation. During the application of spinal manipulation, the practitioner physically moves the spinal joints to restore normal balanced movement. These precise maneuvers are performed by hand and normally produce no pain or discomfort for the patient.

Instability: Cause and Effect

Degenerative disc disease, already explained, results in an unstable segment (or segments). This instability, or shimmy, creates soreness at the ligamentous attachments and causes reactive tension and soreness in the muscles, which are trying to reduce the movement.

Spinal fusion is an operation that eliminates movement between two joints. It is performed in certain cases of severe disc dysfunction. Two to five years after *successful* surgery, however, individuals usually experience secondary back pain. That happens because the joints above and below the fusion become hypermobile, causing the inevitable compensatory soreness of the ligaments and the pain of muscle spasm.

A *sacroiliac joint fixation* similarly will cause compensatory movement, instability, and pain at the opposite sacroiliac joint. Fixation of both sacroiliac joints will cause excessive movement and pain at the adjacent joint (lumbar 5/sacrum1), with probable disability there as well.

The point to remember here is that nature will *always* try to restore normal movement. Where there is any kind of fixation, hypermobility will occur in the adjacent joints. The problem, of course, is that this particular dysfunction — lack of movement combined with compensatory movement — produces a back vulnerable to future pain and disability.

The Back Power Model: A Framework for Management

As we have seen, in dysfunction joints may be (1) locked and immobile or (2) loose, with a shimmy. Muscles may be (1) short and weak or (2) long and weak.

To make sense of all this, we have created what we call the Back Power model (figure 4.5). This model provides a framework for helping us understand how to restore function to the spine.

FIG. 4.5 THE BACK POWER MODEL

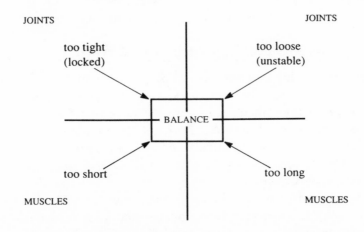

For example, if a joint is fixed and immobile, the appropriate treatment is to restore movement through mobilization, manipulation, or adjustment. If a joint is hypermobile with a shimmy, the appropriate treatment is to restore normal movement through an external support, muscular strength, or, rarely, surgery.

The appropriate treatment for short, weak muscles is to lengthen them through yoga or stretch-relaxation exercises. Long, weak muscles must conversely be tightened through weight lifting or power exercise.

Treating the Spine:
Disease Approach vs. Functional Approach

The two approaches to treating the spine differ in three main ways. First, the disease approach usually focuses on one cause at a specific level in the spine. The functional approach considers dysfunctions of the bones, ligaments, and muscles *at all levels of the trunk or spine.*

A second major difference is that when a disease is found, there will be a definite treatment and prognosis indicated. With dysfunction, there may be three or four (or more) actual dysfunctions to be found, so the approach is more empirical — to try to restore *all* toward normal function. At the same time, it is essential to recognize that the pain symptom usually results from the cumulative effect of the several dysfunctions, not from any one in itself.

The final distinction is that the disease approach is always to "go in and fix the problem." In the functional approach, the key — for practitioner and patient — is to accept what you can't change but change what you can. In certain cases, this means that, realistically, some measure of discomfort or dysfunction may remain residual.

The Biomechanical Approach: A Last Word

Those health professionals who specialize in biomechanical examination of the low back — chiropractors, osteopaths, kinesiologists, physiotherapists — use a wide array of tests to determine minute changes in function. It is not the purpose of this book to describe how and why particular tests are done, only to underscore the fact that the methods are those of functional assessment and, in most cases, produce excellent results.

What we do want to emphasize here is how, by using this functional approach, you can help both yourself and your own health professionals to *manage* your spinal problems by rectifying the biomechanical dysfunctions that are contributing to them.

The next chapter will show you how to begin self-assessment of spine problems — or potential problems — by way of the Back Power tests.

THE BACK POWER PROGRAM

5

The Back Power Tests

This chapter explains how you can assess your own low back function by means of the Back Power tests.

Health professionals have developed many sophisticated tests to measure low back function and discover low back disease. We use these measures to determine a course of therapy and to gauge improvement. But to broaden our focus on pain, treatment, and disease to include fitness, management, and function, we must provide you with tools that you can apply easily to measure low back (dys)function. These will assist you in management of the problem as you pursue better health.

Let's first review the low back's support system. As we have seen, the three basic types of support are:
• muscle support,
• ligamentous support, and
• bony elements (the vertebrae and discs).

Muscles are dynamic and readily amenable to testing and fitness improvement. Ligaments and bony elements are static and much more difficult for personal management. Although improvement in muscular support is primarily a personal responsibility, improvement of joints can be only a health professional's responsibility.

The Pain Factor

It is important to realize that in the low back, dysfunction and pain are not synonymous: you can have a high degree of dysfunction without experiencing pain. Conversely, the presence of pain does always imply dysfunction or disease.

69

If we use the heart attack analogy, we see that dysfunction takes the form of hardening or narrowing of the arteries over many years. This condition will eventually cause the major occlusion (blockage) of the blood vessels — the symptom of pain — that we call a heart attack.

In the same way, your back can be dysfunctional over a number of years, though you may not be aware of the problem. With low back dysfunction, the cumulative effect can be a bout of back pain that may be acute. When the pain settles down, it will leave your back weakened and much more prone to another problem or attack. We call this the disease process. Recurrent bouts of back pain are usually in-terspersed with asymptomatic pain-free episodes.

Before You Begin

If you have had a back problem in the past or if you already prac-tice an exercise regimen, how can you determine when to carry on with your self-help/maintenance or management and when to seek professional help or advice about your back? Let us stress that if you experience back pain, it is most important first to seek professional advice. Although we know that in the majority of cases back pain is caused by *biomechanical dysfunction* (chapters 3 and 4), a professional examination is needed to determine the presence or absence of disease or whether there is an indication that surgery is required.

Next are the two screening tests that we have developed: a questionnaire and a chair test. These must be taken before proceeding to any of the Back Power exercises. Although most people can do the Back Power *tests* without risk, anyone with past or present back problems should have special guidance in the *exercise* program to minimize the risk of recurrent pain.

Back Fitness Questionnaire

If you answer yes to any of these questions, seek professional guidance before attempting the Back Power tests and proceeding to the Back Power exercises:

	Yes	No
• Do you presently suffer from acute back pain?	☐	☐
• Are you currently receiving treatment for back pain?	☐	☐
• Have you had a surgical operation on your back?	☐	☐
• Are you receiving treatment for any serious medical ailment? (e.g., heart condition)	☐	☐
• Has a health professional ever told you never to exercise your back?	☐	☐

The Chair Test

What It Tells You

This test helps to identify an important subgroup of chronic back problems: individuals with a pelvic ring dysfunction. These people can respond poorly to a full Back Power exercise regimen, and they need help desperately. Avoiding exercise is not the answer. The key is to recognize the problem and modify the reconditioning exercises.

If you have difficulty doing the chair test, then you've tested "positive," which means you'll need special and enhanced guidance (see chapter 6) before you undertake the Back Power exercises. You may at first also need professional supervision with the exercises. This means modifying the exercise regimen and metering progressive exercise more carefully.

How To Do It

Stand in front of a normal dining chair (the top of the seat will be about 18 inches from the floor) with your feet flat on the floor and about 6 inches apart. The calves of your legs should be just touching the frame of the chair seat. Now fold your arms across your chest and *slowly* sit down in the chair, making sure to keep your body perfectly vertical as you do so and your feet flat on the floor, still 6 inches apart. You should be able to lower your body slowly into the chair, with your back remaining vertical. You should then be able to rise up slowly from the chair, arms still folded across your chest, feet flat and in the same position on the floor, holding the same vertical position of your back, without dipping forward or jumping up. A successful test (figure 5.1) means that you've sat down and stood up slowly with a perfectly straight back.

FIG. 5.1   CHAIR TEST – NORMAL

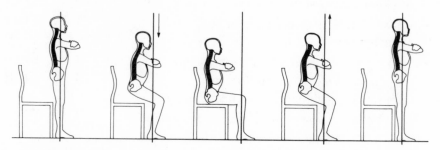

An abnormal or positive test (figure 5.2) means that you've bent your body forward as you sat down and/or you've suddenly sunk or collapsed into the chair at the end of the maneuver. In standing up, you've had to swing forward and/or jump your body up from the chair.

FIG. 5.2   CHAIR TEST – ABNORMAL

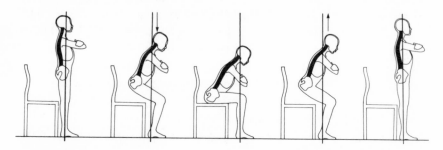

Interpreting Your Results

A positive test usually means that you have a dysfunction of the pelvic ring — the support mechanism for the lumbar spine. If you test positive, you should familiarize yourself with further tests for pelvic ring dysfunction and for a graduated pre-exercise program. These appear in chapter 6. Refer to that chapter before proceeding with any of the Back Power tests, the extension test, or the flexion test.

Not Sure?   If you're not sure about your results in this test, have a friend hold your elbows to make certain you stay vertical and that you go down slowly with your feet remaining flat on the floor. If you still flop into the chair, the test is positive. Next, have your friend keep hold of your elbows as you try to rise from the chair. If you cannot rise slowly, your back straight, feet flat on the floor and 6 inches apart, then your test is positive.

Precautions

There are no precautions to observe for this test. No harm can come to anyone from trying it. As with any test, however, follow the instructions carefully. If you test positive, refer to chapter 6 before reading further.

The Back Power Tests

> **Before beginning each of the four Back Power tests, read complete instructions.**

Who Should Try Them

Who should try the Back Power tests? Everyone!

With approximately 80 percent of the population suffering from back pain at some time in their lives, everyone should try the Back Power tests. These tests, which determine whether low back weakness or dysfunction is present, are the first steps in preventing future problems.

Try the tests:

If you have ever had a bout of acute back pain. Remember, although your pain may have gone, that does not mean you're better. You almost certainly now have mechanical back weakness, and you can benefit from reconditioning exercises.

If you have chronic discomfort and stiffness. You know you have a back problem. With an okay from your health professional, you can derive great benefit from the Back Power tests and exercises.

If you are recovering from acute pain or surgery. With professional guidance you'll find that the tests and exercises will help you to be the best you can be and achieve the best recovery possible for you.

If you suffer from a herniated disc, ankylosing spondylitis, or spondylolisthesis, or have recently recovered from fracture. You can only benefit by strengthening the soft tissue supports of your back — the muscles and ligaments — in order to be the best you can be; but first get clearance from your health professional.

We often say that weak bones supported by weak muscles are a sure recipe for trouble. On the other hand, weak bones supported by strong, balanced muscles eliminate or at least *manage* your problem.

How To Score Them

These four tests evolved from the National Back Fitness Test, which has been used for more than a decade by thousands of people in countless organizations throughout the world. Each test has four levels, with a point score given for each level. Scoring is similar to golf — the lower, the better:

Excellent 1
Good   2
Fair   3
Poor   4

An excellent overall score on the four tests is a total of 4 points. A poor score is 16 points.

Sit-Up Test

What It Tells You
This test measures the suppleness or flexibility of the spine.

How To Do It
Lie on your back on the floor, hands beside you neck and knees bent to a 45° angle to the floor (figure 5.3). Slowly and deliberately, raise your back and shoulders off the floor to a sitting position without jumping or swinging your arms to assist. If you can do this without difficulty, your grade is excellent. *Score 1 point.*

If you can't do the test this way, try again, this time folding your arms across your chest and slowly rising to a sitting position. If this works for you, your score is good. *Score 2 points.*

If you still can't sit up, put your arms straight out in front of you, always keeping your feet flat on the floor, and raise yourself slowly to the sitting position. If you succeed this time, you are fair. *Score 3 points.*

If you can't sit up at all, your score is poor. *Score 4 points.*

Precautions
(1) *Do not* put your hands behind your neck and use your arms and neck to assist you to sit up. This may cause discomfort in your neck and will also give you a false score. (2) *Do not* tuck your feet under an object (e.g., the front of a sofa) or have someone hold your feet down.

Most people can sit up with their feet held, but this version is a different test and does not show back flexibility; rather, it tests the strength of the hip flexors and leg muscles. Doing the test this way would also give you a false score.

FIG. 5.3 **SIT-UP TEST**

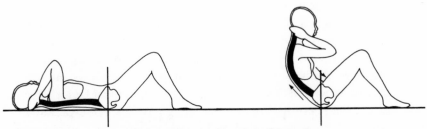

SCORE 1 Able to sit up with knees bent and hands beside neck.

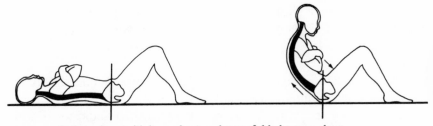

SCORE 2 Able to sit up with knees bent and arms folded across chest.

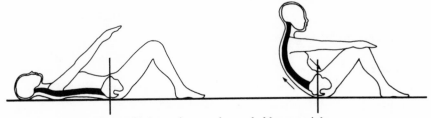

SCORE 3 Able to sit up with knees bent and arms held out straight.

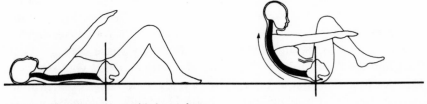

SCORE 4 Unable to sit up with knees bent.

Interpreting Your Results

Many people initially think the sit-up is a test for the stomach muscles or the hip flexors. Indeed, these are the prime movers that pull your body up to the sitting position. The stomach muscles initiate the movement of the head and shoulders off the floor and, as the body rises, the hip flexors take over and complete the movement of a sit-up.

This test, however, though requiring strength in the stomach and sling muscles, is really one of balance between the heavy weight of the head, shoulders, and chest, and the lesser weight of the knees and legs. The only way you can complete a sit-up is if your back is flexible enough to keep the heavy upper body bent in and thus move the center of gravity downward as the sit-up proceeds. The critical factor is back flexibility, which permits stomach and sling muscles to elevate the upper torso. A practical illustration of this balancing is a seesaw: in order to balance, an adult (heavier) with a child (lighter) on the other end would have to move closer to the fulcrum, or center pivot point. In the same way, good back flexibility permits your heavier upper body weight to move closer to the fulcrum of the movement, allowing you to sit up.

One of the earliest signs of low back dysfunction is inflexibility of the spinal joints, which causes stiffness or tightness in the low back muscles. A poor score on this test is a very sensitive indicator of low back dysfunction.

Straight (Double) Leg Raise Test

What It Tells You

This test measures the strength of your stomach muscles by testing their ability to stabilize the trunk under a load.

How To Do It

Lie on your back on the floor, knees bent to a 45° angle, feet flat on the floor, one hand beside your neck. Place your other hand in the hollow between your low back and the floor. Push your back tightly against your hand so that there is no longer any space between your back and the floor. Holding this position tightly by using your stomach muscles to stabilize your back, raise one leg, extending it out straight so that it is about 6 inches off the floor. Hold this position while you check that your back is still tight to the floor. Now raise and extend both legs out straight so that they are about 6 inches off the floor, still keeping your back tight to the floor.

If your back begins to curve away from the floor, stop the test at once. The curving back is arrested by impingement of the facet joints. If held for the full 10 count, discomfort can result.

If you can hold your back tightly on the floor for a count of 10, your score is excellent. *Score 1 point.* If your back is tight at first, then curves away, *score 2 points* for a good score. If your back arches off the floor immediately as your legs are raised, stop the test and take a fair grade of *3 points*. If you can't raise your legs at all, your grade is poor at *4 points*.

FIG. 5.4 **STRAIGHT (DOUBLE) LEG RAISE TEST**

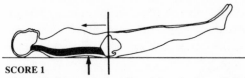

SCORE 1
Able to hold position while raising the legs 6" for a count of 10.

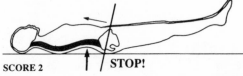

SCORE 2 STOP!
Able to raise the legs for several counts but back curves partway through the test.

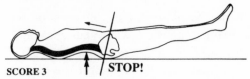

SCORE 3 STOP!
Able to lift the legs but back curves immediately when the legs are raised.

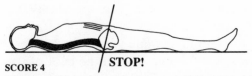

SCORE 4 STOP!
Unable to lift both legs for 10 count and/or lifting legs causes discomfort.

THIS IS NOT AN EXERCISE!
IF YOUR BACK STARTS TO CURVE, STOP!

Precautions

(1) The main precaution is to stop the test the moment your back curves off the floor. When this happens, your back is being limited by the delicate facet joints. This bone-on-bone contact *can* produce injury. (2) Also note that this is a *test* to be *done once. It is not an exercise* to strengthen stomach muscles. In fact, it would be a very poor choice for anyone as an exercise — especially for anyone with a weak back.

Interpreting Your Results

Many people at first think this is a test of sling (hip flexor) muscles, not stomach muscles. It is true that sling muscles are the prime movers of the straight legs, but this is not the movement being tested here. You're testing the ability of your stomach muscles to stabilize your back against the floor and resist the weight of your raised legs. The stronger your stomach muscles, the better you can stabilize your back under mechanical-loading stress (e.g., lifting).

Sling Test

What It Tells You

This test measures the flexibility or length of your sling muscles.

How To Do It

Lie on your back on the floor, hands beside your head, knees bent to a 45° angle, feet flat on the floor. Bring one knee toward your chest and, if you can, hold it tightly against your chest. *Do not raise your chest up to meet your knee.* (If you feel tightening before getting your knee to your chest, *do not force your leg/knee to this position*; instead, add an extra point to your score.) Now, holding your knee to your chest, lower the other leg slowly toward the floor until it is stopped by the tight sling muscles.

If you can hold your knee to your chest while your other leg goes freely down to the floor, *score 1 point* — excellent. If the back of the knee of your extended leg is 2 to 4 inches off the floor, *score 2 points* for a good score; *score 3 points* for 4 to 8 inches off the floor. And if that knee is more than 8 inches off the floor, your score is poor at *4 points*. Remember to add a point if you can't keep your knee tightly against your chest.

FIG. 5.5 SLING TEST

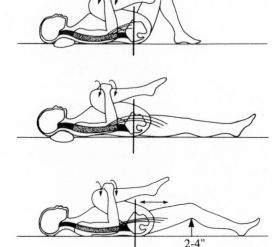

STARTING POSITION

SCORE 1
Able to hold one leg firmly
against the chest with the
other leg flat against the floor.

SCORE 2
With effort able to hold
one knee against the chest
while straightening the
other leg flat to the floor.

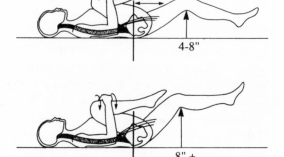
2-4"

SCORE 3
With one knee fixed firmly
against the chest the other
leg will not reach floor.

4-8"

SCORE 4
Unable to get one leg
firmly against the chest
without causing pain or
discomfort and/or other
leg raises off floor
significantly.

8" +

Now, repeat the test with the other leg, noting if there is more tightness on one side than on the other. Note also that when you bring your
right knee to your chest, you are actually measuring the sling muscles
on your *left side*; when you bring your *left knee* to your chest, you are
measuring the *right side* sling muscles.

To arrive at your final score on this test, add the scores for left and
right legs and divide by two for the average. For example, *4 points* on
one side plus *2 points* on the other add up to *6*; divide by two for a
score of *3 points*.

Precautions

(1) If your knee does not come tightly to your chest, take *1 point off* your score but *do not force your knee to your chest*. This move can produce strain of the muscles or joints. (2) *Do not force your leg down to the floor.* This move also can strain muscles or joints and must be avoided. (In addition, it would give an unrealistic score and defeat the purpose of the test.) (3) If you have painful or injured knees, you can do this test by placing your hands *behind* your knee on your thigh. (4) If you have hip disease with limited hip range of movement, you may not get a proper score on this test.

Interpreting Your Results

If in either case you are unable to lower your leg smoothly to the floor, the sling muscles being tested are tight and weak and in need of stretching.

Lateral Lift Test

What It Tells You

The lateral lift tests the strength of the lateral (side) muscles.

How To Do It

A partner is needed to assist with this test. Lie on one side with your arms folded across your chest. Your body should be extended full length in a straight line. Your partner must lean on your ankles so that they are firmly held to the floor. Then, keeping your body straight — no twisting — raise your shoulder as high as possible up off the floor. Hold the position, and measure the distance between the low side of your shoulder and the floor. This move must be a pure lift, held for a moment, and then repeated for the other side of your body by lying on the opposite side.

If you can raise your shoulders 12 inches or more off the floor, you have an excellent score at *1 point*. From 6 to 12 inches is good at *2 points*. From 2 to 6 inches is a fair score at *3 points*. If you can't raise your shoulders at all or can raise them less than 2 inches, you have a poor score at *4 points*.

As you did for the previous test, add your score from each side and divide by two for the average, or final score.

FIG. 5.6 LATERAL LIFT TEST

SCORE 1
Able to raise the shoulders
12" off the floor without
difficulty.

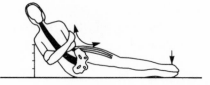

SCORE 2
Able to raise the shoulders
6-12" off the floor but with
difficulty.

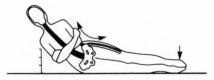

SCORE 3
Able to raise shoulders 2-6"
off the floor with difficulty.

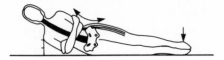

SCORE 4
Unable to raise shoulders
off the floor.

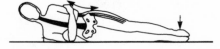

Precautions
(1) Do not jump or flip your body up. (2) Do not twist your body. (3) Do not push off with your elbow.

Interpreting Your Results
This test indicates the strength of the lateral muscles of the trunk, the hip, and the leg.

Two Other Tests for Measuring Flexibility

In order to provide an overall measure of total range of spine movement, we incorporate two other tests, the extension test and the flexion test.

Before taking the extension and flexion tests, read complete instructions.

Extension Test

What It Tells You
This test assesses back flexibility in a direct way, requiring no muscular action at all.

How To Do It
Lie on your stomach on the floor and place your hands under your shoulders, as if you were going to do a push-up. Instead, just push your chest away from the floor so that your shoulders come up but your pelvis/hip bones remain on the ground. (You may have to practice this once or twice.) When taking this test, you should be perfectly limp, with no muscle contraction in your back. If necessary, have a partner hold your pelvis over the tail bone and tell you to stop when the tail bone starts to lift. Measure the distance between the floor and the notched bone (the sternal notch) at the front base of the neck.

If you can extend by 12 inches or more, *score 1 point*. This is excellent. For 8 to 12 inches, *score 2 points*, for good. Fair is 4 to 8 inches, *scoring 3 points*. Under 4 inches is poor, for *1 point*.

FIG. 5.7 **EXTENSION TEST**

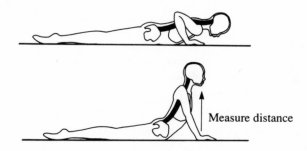

Measure distance

Precautions
(1) Stop the test if pain occurs; don't push further. This usually means that you're jamming your facet joints together. (2) Do not let your pelvis rise off the floor; this move would make for an unrealistic score. (3) Do not be competitive. This is a test to help you assess your function, not impress your friends.

Interpreting Your Results
A good to excellent score indicates a flexible back. A poor score indicates low back dysfunction.

Flexion Test

What It Tells You
This test measures the total forward overall movement of your spine.

How To Do It
Sit on the floor with your legs straight out in front and ankles at 90°. Stretch your arms forward toward your toes until you are stopped by tightness or discomfort in the back or legs. *Do not overstretch.*

If you can reach well past your toes, *score 1 point* for an excellent score. Reaching just to the toes is good for *2 points*. Up to 4 inches from the toes is fair, for *3 points*. More than 4 inches away is poor, for *4 points*.

FIG. 5.8 FLEXION TEST

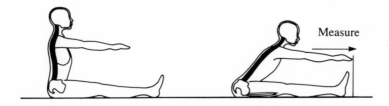

Precautions
Stop when you feel tightness or discomfort in your back or leg.

Interpreting Your Results.
Fair or poor results (*3 to 4 points*) on this test indicate loss of total back flexibility as well as loss of hamstring muscle flexibility.

You can measure *total back flexibility* by regularly applying the extension and flexion tests.

How Strong Is Your Back?

The Four Back Power Tests — Interpreting Your Total Score

Taking your scores from the four Back Power tests (sit-up; straight leg raise; sling test; lateral lift test), a total ranging from *4* (excellent) to *16* (poor) is possible.

A total of 4 or 5 is excellent. If your total is 5, you should be able to attain a perfect score with little difficulty.

A total of 6 to 8 is good, but you still need to do some work to stretch and strengthen your trunk muscles.

A total of 9 to 10 is fair and means you have quite a lot of work to do to get your trunk muscles into better shape through stretching-strengthening exercises. You *may* require some professional guidance.

A total over 10 means that you have a lot of work to do. You *may* require professional help.

6

Pelvic Ring Dysfunction: Special Tests

The Vital Connector

We earlier referred to the pelvic ring as the "vital connector." Its function is to link the spine — the body's major weight-transmitting structure — to the ground via the legs and feet. The three bones of the pelvic ring (the sacrum and the two hip bones) form five joints: the two sacroiliac joints, the two hip joints, and the symphysis pubis. (This is shown in chapter 3, figure 3.8.)

Figure 6.1 illustrates the coupling effect of the joints of the pelvic ring. This *pelvic couple* acts as a spring, tightening up and forming a

FIG. 6.1 THE FUNCTIONING PELVIS

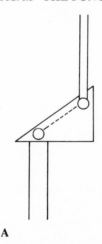 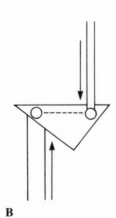 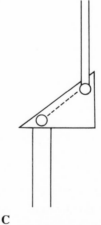

A

Pelvic ring uncoupled

B

Pelvic ring coupled (locked) bearing weight

C

Pelvic ring restored to uncoupled position

self-locking mechanism for stability when weight-bearing comes into play. In the movement/flexibility mode, with weight removed, this mechanism becomes looser and more flexible, permitting mobility for normal walking and running movement.

As illustrated in figure 6.2, the pelvic couple is also acted on by the four types of trunk muscles *above* the pelvic ring (the back, stomach, sling, and lateral muscles); and, *below* the pelvic ring, by the quadriceps (muscles at front of thighs) and hamstrings (those in back of thighs).

FIG. 6.2 MUSCLES ACTING ON THE PELVIC RING

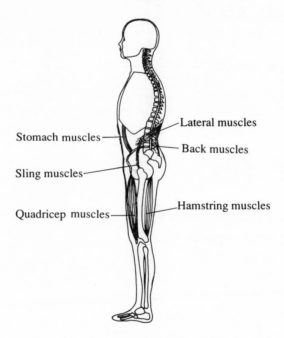

Stomach muscles

Sling muscles

Quadricep muscles

Lateral muscles

Back muscles

Hamstring muscles

Our typical patient with pain caused by a pelvic ring dysfunction will arrive limping. Asked to localize the pain, he or she will put a hand over the sacroiliac area, sometimes also indicating that the pain in that area radiates down into the leg. (Pain that radiates this way is usually experienced in the thigh, rarely traveling below the knee.)

People with pelvic ring disorders have trouble climbing stairs and difficulty getting into or out of a chair, usually having to push themselves up from a sitting position by using their arms. An intertrochanteric belt often relieves their pain dramatically and improves their function in both stair climbing and getting out of a chair. (This belt is described in detail at the end of this chapter.)

Examination of the hip area usually reveals tight, fibrositic trigger points or nodules in the muscles there. In general, the pain caused by pelvic ring disorder is very resistant to conventional treatment, taking from three to six months to settle down properly — if at all. And the problem has a very high risk of recurrence.

The Sacroiliac Controversy

No other joint in the body has been the subject of as much controversy as the sacroiliac joint.

In North America, the traditional view among surgeons has been that sacroiliac joints do not move and that they are not a source of low back pain.* In Europe, however, orthopedic surgeons and specialists do accept that sacroiliac joints can be a source of pain. And, as a group, the practitioners who deal with hands-on treatment of the hip and back areas are quite adamant that sacroiliac joints do become unstable and/or fixed, and that they do create low back disorders.

The Obstetricians' View

If we look at studies on the subject, we discover that obstetricians in particular describe problems in the pelvic ring and sacroiliac area — and with good reason.

In the later months of pregnancy, many women develop pain in the low back and hips — specifically, over the sacroiliac joints. These women are thought to have unstable sacroiliac joints because the high level of hormones in their system at this stage of pregnancy causes a loosening of the ligaments that join the sacroiliac joints. Because the baby has to be delivered through the pelvic ring and pelvic channel, this is a most welcome phenomenon: the hormonal influence that has loosened the ligaments has created an easier passage for the body and head of the baby. For obvious reasons, women who

---

* Dr. Ian Macnab, however, one of North America's most esteemed orthopedic surgeons, not only describes sacroiliac joints as a source of pain but recommends an intertrochanteric belt as a source of relief (in his book *Backache*, Baltimore: Williams & Wilkins, 1977).

have this loose pelvic ring condition tend to deliver their babies very quickly.

On the negative side, many women who develop this loosening of ligaments may not recover healthy ligamentous tightness after their pregnancies. Instead, they are often left with chronic low back pain or a weakened back susceptible to injury.

Diagnosis: A Special Problem

O ne of the major impediments to accepting the idea that sacroiliac joints are the source of problems is that of diagnosis: it is extremely difficult to determine whether these joints are healthy or ailing.

Where pain is present in the *sacroiliac syndrome*, it is usually located in the region of the sacroiliac joint with or without referred pain in the groin on the same side. Pain may also be referred to the buttock or down the back of the leg to the knee or in the front of the thigh. The leg may feel heavy or weak and is usually aggravated by rising from a chair after prolonged sitting.

Motion-palpation studies are among the most common methods used to test for function in the sacroiliac joints. The examiner places one thumb on the patient's sacrum (tail bone), then the other on the hip (innominate) bone. The patient must then raise one knee up toward the chest. This action causes certain normal and abnormal movements to take place. Motion-palpation studies can, however, be inconsistent as a test.

Sacroiliac Studies

A great deal of work on sacroiliac joints has been done by Dr. David Cassidy, a chiropractor who has been working for ten years with Dr. Kirkaldy-Willis, a prominent orthopedic surgeon, at the University Hospital in Saskatoon, Saskatchewan. Kirkaldy-Willis and Cassidy found that sacroiliac joints do in fact move — but not very much. What happens at the sacroiliac joint is a gliding, which permits people to walk and allows flexibility and movement in locomotion.

If the sacroiliac joints are too tight, however, walking tends to have a peculiar wiggle around the axis of the spine, which in turn often causes problems and inordinate movement at the L5/S1 disc.

People with very lax sacroiliac joints on both sides tend to waddle — a condition often seen in women who have had numerous pregnancies. As they walk, their hips go up and down, in much the same way as the pistons on a steam locomotive.

Studies have shown that in children the sacroiliac joints do have significant movement. Then, as we mature, the movement becomes less and less until in old age the sacroiliac joints are usually fused. Along the way, however, abnormal changes or dysfunction can occur. We'll look at these shortly in our description of the four types of disorders that occur in pelvic ring dysfuntion.

Detecting Pelvic Ring Dysfunction

The Chair test (see chapter 5) is a simple way to detect pelvic ring dysfunction.

Try this test again and make a mental note of how far your body bends forward to maintain balance during descent *into* and ascent *out of* the chair. Now apply an intertrochanteric belt (see the end of this chapter).

Once the belt is in place, make sure it extends over your hip bones and around the midpoint of your buttocks. It must be tight enough that one finger can just get in between the belt and your skin.

Now try the chair test again (figure 6.3).

FIG. 6.3 **CHAIR TEST FOR PELVIC DYSFUNCTION IMPROVED WITH INTERTROCHANTERIC BELT**

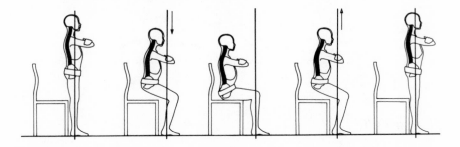

For some of you, the belt will be a dream come true: you'll be able to sit down easily with your body erect and practically float up out of the chair when you stand, with no difficulty at all. If this happens for you, follow the procedure for a *Type 1* pelvic ring disorder, described later in this chapter.

If, however the belt does not make much difference or if it worsens your performance of the Chair test, you should try the following tests for muscle balance.

Testing Your Muscle Balance

Quad (Thigh) Test

What It Tells You
The quad test measures the length of the *quadriceps* (thigh muscles). These are the muscles that run down the front of your thighs to your kneecaps.

How To Do It
Lie on your stomach with your legs stretched out. Swing your right arm back and bend your right knee, bringing your heel toward your buttocks. Grasp the foot in your hand, pulling your heel forward until the muscles start to get tight. Measure the distance between the top of your buttocks and the back of your heel. This indicates the length of your quadricep in the right thigh. Now test your left leg in the same way. Record both measurements. Are the measures the same, or does one heel come in more tightly than the other?

FIG. 6.4   QUAD (THIGH) TEST

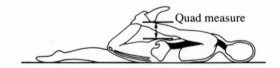

Hamstring Test

What It Tells You
This test measures the hamstrings, which are the muscles in the back of your legs, running from your pelvis to your knees. If you place your hand in this area while sitting in a chair and push your heel against a leg of the chair, you should feel the hamstring muscle contract and tighten.

How To Do It

Sit on the floor, legs straight out, then bring one foot up and place it opposite the other knee. Now bend forward, bringing your forehead as close as you can to the knee of the leg that is still straight out. Measure the distance between your forehead and the top of that knee. Repeat with the other leg. Record both measurements, noting difference.

FIG. 6.5 HAMSTRING TEST

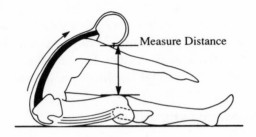

Measure Distance

Glut (Buttock) Test

What It Tells You

This test measures the *gluteal* (buttock) muscles. If you put your hand on your buttock and tighten the muscles there, you'll be able to feel the gluteals contract.

How To Do It

Lie on your back on the floor, legs straight out. Put the toes of one foot under the back of the knee of the opposite leg, bending your knee and grasping it with the opposite hand, as illustrated in figure 6.6. Now roll that knee sideways until it is limited by a feeling of tightness or discomfort in the gluteal muscles. Repeat this maneuver on the other side and record whether one side feels significantly tighter than the other.

FIG. 6.6 GLUT (BUTTOCK) TEST STRETCH-RELAXATION

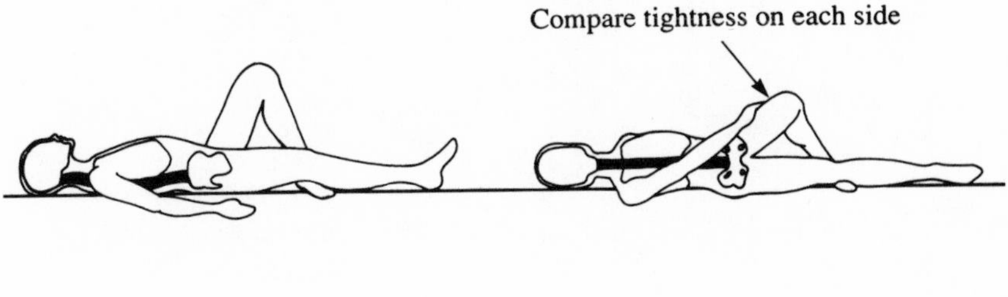

Compare tightness on each side

Pelvic Ring Disorders

Which type of pelvic ring disorder is affecting you?

Type 1 Disorder

This disorder (figure 6.7) occurs in women who have been pregnant, and particularly in those who have been pregnant a number of times. Type 1 disorder occurs because the high level of hormones during the latter months of pregnancy causes an increase in elasticity of the strong ligaments joining the hip bones to the sacrum. Delivery of the baby further loosens these ligaments. In the Type 1 disorder, the normal ligamentous tension and function are not restored.

FIG. 6.7 **PELVIC RING DISORDER: TYPE 1**

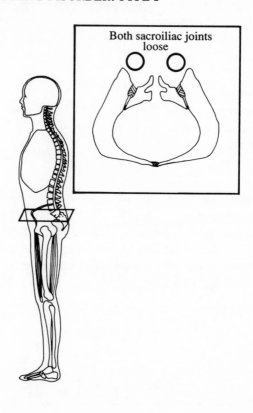

Both sacroiliac joints loose

Women experiencing this disorder often complain of pain over *both* sacroiliac areas and may walk with a waddle.

In the Type 1 disorder, thigh muscles, hamstrings, and buttock muscles are usually loose. There is very little muscular tightness.

Management of this disorder includes wearing a tight intertrochanteric belt for two to three weeks. In rare instances, the belt may have to be worn for longer than three weeks.

At any recurrence of pain, the belt should be worn for a few days. It may also be used as an aid when lifting or moving furniture or other heavy objects.

In addition to doing the Back Power exercises described in the following chapter, those with Type 1 pelvic ring disorder should place particular emphasis on increasing the strength of the stomach and lateral muscles. You should *avoid the sling stretch exercise*: it can sometimes cause loosening of the ligaments as the muscles are being stretched. Exercise strategy for the Type 1 disorder is outlined in table 6.1.

TABLE 6.1

Exercise Strategy for Type 1 Pelvic Ring Disorder

Test	*Muscle Tested*	*Exercise*
Sit-Up	Back flexibility	Mad Cat
Straight Leg Raise	Stomach strength	**Curl/Sit-Down** ✖
Sling Test	Sling flexibility	Sling Stretch ✖
Lateral Lift Test	Lateral flexibility and strength	Side Stretch **Lateral Lift**

USE BELT INITIALLY DURING EXERCISES

> **Bold type means emphasize this exercise**
> ✖   means avoid this exercise

Type 2 Disorder

This pelvic ring disorder (figure 6.8) is the opposite condition of Type 1.

In the Type 2 disorder, both sacroiliac joints are fused and are tight. Type 2 can happen in young people — especially men — as part of ankylosing spondylitis, the inflammatory arthritis that commonly localizes to one or both sacroiliac joints. Type 2 may also occur as one of the more natural phenomena of aging.

FIG. 6.8 PELVIC RING DISORDER: TYPE 2

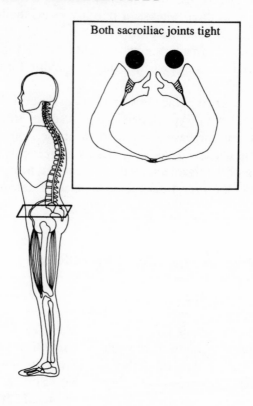

Whatever the cause, the net result of this condition is an alteration in normal smooth walking, often producing a horizontal wiggle as opposed to the vertical waddle of Type 1. In addition, this tightness produces excessive movement and biomechanical strains in the L5/S1 and L4/L5 disc areas.

The quadriceps, hamstrings, and buttock muscles are usually loose in this disorder. Should they be tight, however, treatment/management requires stretching these muscles. Exercise strategy for the Type 2 disorder is outlined in Table 6.2.

TABLE 6.2

Exercise Strategy for Type 2 and 3 Pelvic Ring Disorders

Pre-Exercise Stretches: *Glut (Buttock) Test*
                                Quad (Thigh) Test
                                Hamstring Test

Test	*Muscle Tested*	*Exercise*
Sit-Up	Back flexibility	**Mad Cat**
Straight Leg Raise	Stomach strength	**Sit-Down**
Sling Test	Sling flexibility	**Sling Stretch** *with care!*
Lateral Lift Test	Lateral flexibility and strength	Side Stretch Lateral Lift

DO NOT USE BELT FOR TYPE 3 DISORDER

> **Bold type means emphasize this exercise**

Type 3 Disorder

This disorder is also characterized by bilateral tightening of the sacroiliac joints and loosening of the associated lumbar 4/5 disc joints. In the Type 3 disorder, however, both quadriceps are extremely tight and usually symmetrical (the same in both legs). In this disorder, the hamstrings and buttock muscles are usually also very tight. Type 3 individuals are often young and extremely athletic; their musclebound quads are actually a product of their sports activities. The Type 3 tight muscular condition causes excessive torquing in each hip bone and a loss of motion in the sacroiliac joints.

Exercise strategy for Type 3 calls for stretching of the quadriceps, hamstrings, and buttock muscles. This stretching is often followed by an instant and dramatic improvement in the Chair test.

Try the stretching exercises described in the next chapter and then take the Chair test again. The results may surprise you. As you persevere with these stretching exercises, your ability to do the Chair test will improve and your back will function more normally, removing mechanical stress from other areas of your back.

The intertrochanteric belt usually only aggravates a Type 3 disorder and should not be used. Exercise strategy for the Type 3 disorder is outlined in table 6.2.

FIG. 6.9   **PELVIC RING DISORDER: TYPE 3**

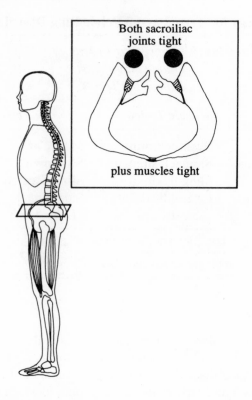

Type 4 Disorder

This type of pelvic ring disorder is probably the most common. Here, tightness of one sacroiliac joint produces a compensatory looseness of the opposite sacroiliac joint. It is the loose joint that is usually painful.

This condition can be caused by jamming or underlying joint pathology but may also be caused by a fall on one hip. It can happen in sports or by slipping or otherwise falling accidentally. There is often an asymmetrical tightening of one quadricep: the tight quad produces fixation on its own side and compensatory hypermobility on the other.

Type 4 individuals are usually quite athletic, but for some reason they are subject to the asymmetrical tightening condition described, rather than to the symmetrical tightening of Type 3 people. Often they manifest leg-length discrepancy.

FIG. 6.10 PELVIC RING DISORDER: TYPE 4

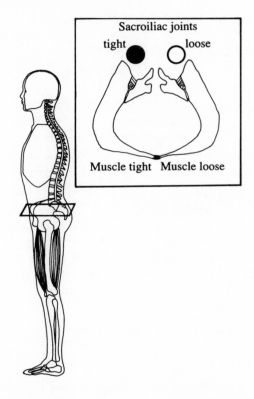

Sacroiliac joints

tight   loose

Muscle tight   Muscle loose

Exercise strategy for Type 4 pelvic ring disorder should include all the thigh, hamstring, and buttock stretches along with the full Back Power exercise program, outlined in the next chapter. Particular emphasis should be placed on strengthening the stomach and lateral muscles and *particular care should be taken* with both the lateral and the sling stretch exercises. Exercise strategy for the Type 4 disorder is outlined in table 6.3.

Hip Joint Disorders

In looking at these four main types of pelvic ring disorder, we have concentrated on the sacroiliac joints. But these are only two of the five joints that make up the pelvic ring, the others being the two hip joints and the symphysis pubis, where the two hip bones join in front.

The *symphysis pubis* rarely causes any problems, except in the case of serious accident and subsequent trauma.

TABLE 6.3

Exercise Strategy for Type 4 Pelvic Ring Disorder

Pre-Exercise Stretches: *Glut (Buttock) Test*
                            Quad (Thigh) Test
                            Hamstring Test

Test	*Muscle Tested*	*Exercise*
Sit-Up	Back flexibility	**Mad Cat**
Straight Leg Raise	Stomach strength	**Sit-Down**
Sling Test	Sling flexibility	Sling Stretch *with care!*
Lateral Lift Test	Lateral flexibility and strength	Side Stretch *with care!* **Lateral Lift**

With Type 4 disorders, it is important to wear an intertrochanteric belt when doing these exercises. Also, special care is required for both Sling Stretch and Lateral Stretch exercises during the first 3-4 weeks of your exercise program.

> Bold type means emphasize this exercise

Occasionally, however, one or both of the *hip joints* become loose, causing a disorder that is very similar to Type 4. An indication of this condition can sometimes be spotted on the lateral lift test (described in the preceding chapter). The hip joint will be seen to rotate excessively. Also, during certain movements or exercises, an individual may hear audible clicks that strongly suggest an instability somewhere in the pelvic ring.

Treatment/management of this condition is the same as Type 4.

Summing Up

Incredible as it may seem, the pelvic ring disorders are often overlooked by doctors whose patients suffer from low back pain. Yet they account for up to 30 percent of the chronic back pain cases seen in our practice. And they are very easily recognized just by the chair test.

Although the pelvic ring disorders are very resistant to normal treatments, with a poor response to rest and a very high rate of recurrence, they can be effectively managed. Where dysfunction is in the form of looseness, the intertrochanteric belt and appropriate exercises combine to help people take control of their lives — and be the best they can be. Where tightness is the problem, joint manipulation together with the right stretching and strengthening exercises are appropriate.

And in prescribing any exercise regimen, it is most important to *recognize* if you have one of the pelvic ring disorders. As we've indicated earlier in this chapter, certain exercises, if carried out without regard to these disorders, can actually increase pain and discourage an individual from continuing. In the Back Power program, these exercises are the *Sling Stretch* and the *Side Stretch*. Both should be done with great care if you have a pelvic ring disorder.

Indeed, when doing any of the exercises that are described in the next chapter, if you experience pain over the sacroiliac joint (s), you should seek professional guidance before continuing. And although these exercises can usually be continued with great benefit, note that if the belt is called for in your type of disorder, it must be worn during the exercise session. This is important because it stabilizes the loose pelvic area while the exercises stretch and strengthen the surrounding muscles.

The next section of this chapter will tell you more about that belt.

The Back Power Belt

Belts, braces, and supports have been used for years to stabilize the spine. Belts have fallen into disfavor in many quarters because of discomfort (they make the wearer hot or "sweaty," chafe the skin, or restrict breathing and activity) and concern about a degree of dysfunction that some belts produce (loss of range of movement, muscle weakness, stiffness).

The Back Power belt was developed over many years by Dr. Lyman Johnston, a skilled chiropractor from Toronto, who has always used his leisure time to experiment with and perfect devices to assist suffering patients. The story goes that on a trip to New York City, Dr. Johnston was walking along the harbor, watching ships being loaded and unloaded. He noticed that the stevedores, when they weren't working, wore a wide belt around their waists. Then, as they resumed their heavy work, the stevedores would adjust their belts down around their hips, tightening them in the process. Dr. Johnston was intrigued. He spoke to some of the men and learned that they felt much more stable for lifting and carrying jobs when these belts were in place.

They also told him that the belt seemed to play a part in limiting the amount of injury the men suffered as a group.

Although a wide belt appears to be a straightforward bit of technology, Lyman Johnston would find himself doing much research and involved in the usual processes of trial and error before perfecting what we now know as the Back Power belt.

Where Is It Worn?

The Back Power belt is an intertrochanteric belt (inter = between; trochanter = hip), worn over your hip bones and circling the pelvic ring. It should be positioned 1½ to 2 inches below the top of the pelvic bone. Thus, the belt reduces excess movement in the five joints that form the foundation of the back (symphysis pubis, hip joints, and sacroiliac joints). If the joints are too tight, the belt will increase the tightness and possibly cause or increase discomfort temporarily. In other types of belts, the stabilization occurs above the pelvis, in the lumbar area. Such belts provide a completely *different* type of support and will not substitute for the Back Power belt or improve performance in the Chair test.

When Is It Worn?

Normally, the belt is worn as long as you have pain in the pelvic ring. It is worn initially in the first few weeks of pelvic ring disorder (especially Type 4) exercises. If you have pelvic ring trouble, wear the belt when lifting or moving heavy objects. We recommend wearing it until the Chair test is normal. The belt is generally worn days and some nights (when you have pain rolling over). It provides support for ligaments and bones, and it does not create muscle weakness.

How Tight?

Another major finding is that the belt must be worn very snugly — so that you should be able to get only one finger between the belt and your body.

Ordinary belts have eyelets, and the space between them permits excessive loosening of the belt and loss of maximum benefit. For this reason, there is an ingenious patented locking device on the Back Power belt that can click tightly in small increments, allowing just the right level of support.

If the belt is *too* tight, you may feel some discomfort in your buttock, indicating interference with circulation. If the belt is placed over a tender area of fibrositis, you may feel some pain in *that* area or referred pain down into the thigh. In either case, simply move the belt slightly up or down and/or loosen it off one notch.

How Is It Worn?

It is most important that the belt resist slipping upward in the activities of daily living. The buckle worn over the left hip helps to resist upward movement as well as prevent pinching when you sit in a chair. Adjustable rubber pads also help prevent slippage. The belt is worn with greatest comfort and least slippage *over* your clothes. When you are in public, you may prefer to wear it over your undergarments, inside your outer clothing.

What Is It Made Of?

The material used in the belt can't stretch. A tightly woven fabric provides constant support and also molds to your individual shape. The belt is 2 to 3 inches wide, to give best support with maximum comfort. Narrower belts cut off the circulation; wider belts become uncomfortable.

How To Make Your Own Belt

1) Measure your hips at their widest diameter.
2) Buy a long, pliable, nonelastic belt that is 2 to 3 inches wide.
3) Before making your own intertrochanteric belt, try the Chair test (chapter 5).
4) Now, place the belt in the intertrochanteric position — about two fingers below the top of your pelvic bone.
5) Tighten the belt snugly around your hips so that only one finger will slip between the belt and you body. The belt must pass over the middle of your buttocks.
6) If there is no eyelet in the belt at the point required, mark the spot where it should be. Then make the eyelet in the belt at a tighter point — about one-quarter inch further in.
7) Place the belt in the proper position again, but this time buckle up.
8) Try the Chair test again.

7

The Back Power and Muscle Maintenance Exercises

Introduction

If you haven't tried the Back Power tests, take a moment to find out your personal back fitness level. Most people are quite surprised how poorly they score. The tests look so simple ("What? Only one sit-up?"), yet only one person in ten will have a score of excellent.

If you are in this fortunate group, you suffer little back discomfort and no doubt keep very active. If you did poorly, you probably belong to that massive group of 80 percent of the population suffering from back problems. The worse your score, the more likely you are to suffer severe back problems. One of these profiles may fit you:

- Individuals with pelvic ring disorders who require a carefully graded, specific reconditioning program.
- Young athletic men and, to a lesser extent, athletic women, who often fare poorly on the tests not because their muscle bulk and tone are poor but because their activity has created a musclebound position of poor muscle flexibility and, thus, weakness.
- The majority of women — they score well on the flexibility tests (sit-up and sling tests) but very poorly on stomach strength.
- Manual workers, who usually score well on stomach strength but, like the athletes (doing a heavy job is being an athlete), usually demonstrate loss of flexibility.
- Individuals with a previous back injury. The old injury will leave one side of the back weak and contracted. In the sling and lateral lift tests, test scores for one side of the body will differ significantly from scores for the other.

• People with scoliosis, who often find a significant asymmetrical muscle imbalance, primarily in the sling and lateral muscle groups.

If your score is poor and you've never had back pain, that's unusual! Perhaps you're just living too sedentary a life-style, or maybe you're just lucky. Don't keep counting on luck. Try the exercises.

The Back Power Program — How It Works

1. Score Yourself on the Back Power Tests (Chapter 5)

2. Develop These Skills:
   • Relaxed Breathing
   • Effective Stretch-Relaxation
   • Pelvic Tilt Position

3. Advance to Back Power Program:

   A.   *Begin with Back Power Exercises**

Exercise	*Type*
Sling-Stretch	Stretch-Relaxation
Mad Cat	Stretch-Relaxation
Side Stretch	Stretch-Relaxation
Sit-Down	Power-Strength
Lateral Lift	Power-Strength

   B.   *When you can do these with ease, add on Muscle Maintenance*

   Shoulder Stretch-Relaxation
   Groin Stretch-Relaxation
   Hamstring Stretch-Relaxation
   Calf Stretch-Relaxation
   Quadricep Stretch-Relaxation
   Power-Strength Push-Up

   * If you received an excellent score on the Back Power Tests, advance directly to the total Back Power Program

---

Emphasize Your Weaknesses

The Back Power tests point out specifically the muscles that are weak because of lack of balance. Although you should do *all* the exercises in the program, you must place special emphasis on your own areas of weakness and need, as determined by your own individual scores on the tests.

Some people like to do exercises they're good at, but that's not the point here. Rather, you must improve and bring your weaknesses up to the same high level as your strengths. *Balance* is the key to a healthy back, just as it is to healthy individual muscle groups.

Stretch-Relaxation and Power-Strength Exercises

In time, you'll become quite comfortable with Back Power's stretch-relaxation and power-strength exercises. When you can do them with ease, it will be time to graduate to Muscle Maintenance, which adds six more exercises: five stretch-relaxation exercises and one power-strength exercise. The combination gives you a complete but simple program, necessary for maintaining strength and balance of your musculature in your trunk, your arms, and your legs.

The *power-strength exercises*, very similar to weight lifting, tighten long muscles to their optimal working length. The *stretch-relaxation* exercises are for muscles that have become
• shortened through stress,
• musclebound from excessive activity,
• contracted through injury and spasm, or
• just tight from age and disuse.
These exercises will restore the muscles' optimal midrange working length.

A Balanced, Powerful Muscle

The whole Back Power/Muscle Maintenance program is based on the muscle power-length principle of muscle physiology. In chapter 4 we described how muscles work and spoke of this power-length relationship. We explained that muscles that are too short or too long are weak, while strong, powerful muscles must be in their balanced midposition. The principle is illustrated in figure 7.1.

A muscle is made up of many muscle fibers. Within these fibers are specialized sensors, called muscle spindles, which determine the length of a muscle and its degree of tone. Muscle spindles help muscles maintain postural balance. If a muscle spindle is stimulated to relax, it will lengthen, permitting the muscle to lengthen. As we'll explain, relaxed breathing is a powerful stimulus that allows muscle

FIG. 7.1 MUSCLE LENGTH-POWER RELATIONSHIP

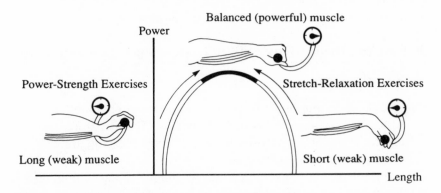

spindles, and thus muscles, to relax; it is an essential skill if you are to be successful with the stretch-relaxation exercises.

If a muscle is *overstretched*, the length of the muscle spindle is exceeded, causing it to "fire off" and the muscle to contract. The results in effect work at cross purposes: an actively contracted muscle *cannot relax*.

Who Needs the Back Power Program?

Who needs the Back Power program? Practically everyone! The spine and trunk are the foundation of our bodies both as a support system and as a firm basis for all movement. Because most people lack strength and fitness in this crucial area, is it any wonder that so many suffer recurrent or chronic low back pain?

Our regimen uses gentle stretching to lengthen tight muscles while balancing joints. Nevertheless, readers with back pain are advised to seek professional advice and guidance before embarking on the program. Your practitioner may advise a slight modification of the exercise program to best meet your specific situation.

What about Specific Disease in the Low Back?

With the exception of *the serious internal medical problem*, Back Power exercises can play a significant role for all conditions: a herniated disc, inflammatory arthritis, spondylolisthesis, a fracture, or a post-surgical situation. We often say:

• Weak joints supported by weak muscles are a sure recipe for future problems.

- Weak joints supported by strong, balanced muscles will eliminate or at least manage you problem.
- Are you willing to be the best you can possible be?

Before You Begin: Three Skills To Develop

Relaxed Breathing

Although breathing is an instinctive act, relaxed breathing is one of the most difficult things to teach people. This is particularly true of athletic males who are used to doing things the "tough" way and subscribe to the "no pain, no gain" philosophy.

Nevertheless, our relaxed breathing technique is an essential part of all the stretch-relaxation exercises that follow. Here's how you do it:

1. Sit in a comfortable chair, arms dangling by your side, head forward with chin on chest and eyes closed.
2. Breathe in deeply, at first allowing the abdomen to expand and then the chest. As you breathe in, your shoulders will rise naturally. Hold your breath for a moment.
3. Now breathe out slowly. Feel your shoulders and arms droop limply. Feel your head passively fall forward and your body become heavy.
4. When your breath has fully expired, your body is completely limp. This is the *maximum relaxation phase*, when muscle spindles are causing your muscles to stretch to their fullest.
5. Now breathe in and repeat the breathing exercise several times. Notice how relaxed your whole body begins to feel.

FIG. 7.2 **RELAXED BREATHING**

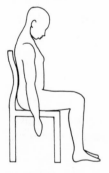 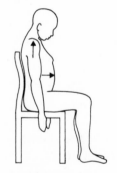 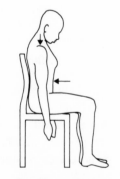

Relax   Breathe in   Breathe out slowly

Effective Stretch-Relaxation

This four-step approach to effective stretch-relaxation is the method we advocate in our exercises.

1. Stretch the muscle in the movement indicated until you feel a "wall" — a place where you have pain or where the muscle will stretch no further. Back off slightly from this position and hold it, maintaining the slightly relaxed length.

2. Now use the relaxed breathing method, taking a deep breath that fills your whole body (described above). Let out the last of that breath.

3. Let your body fully and consciously relax.

4. Take up slack in the muscle by stretching it gently until you feel a new point of resistance — a new "wall." Stop stretching, back off a little, and repeat the stretching process until the muscle lets you go no further or until you feel discomfort.

The Pelvic Tilt Position

The pelvic tilt is the basic posture held during the Back Power exercises. It is essential to learn this position because once you've adopted it, you minimize risk to your back. As we've seen in earlier chapters, your back is at its strongest when it is in the balanced pelvic position. That is because your spine is straighter, more neutral. The more curved the spine, the more susceptible it is to injury.

Here are two methods to help you actually *feel* the pelvic tilt:

Standing
1. Stand with your back and buttocks against a wall.
2. Place your hands between the small of your back and the wall.
3. Place one foot on a chair seat in front of you.
4. Now, notice how your pelvis is tilted up and your back is straighter and nearer to the wall than it was when both feet were on the ground. *This is the pelvic tilt position.*

Lying Down
1. Lie on your back, with knees bent at the angle shown in figure 7.3.
2. Place your hand between the small of your back and the floor.
3. Flatten your back against your hand and the floor by contracting your stomach muscles and rotating your hips backward.

4. Breathe out deeply. *This is the pelvic tilt position.*

FIG. 7.3 THE PELVIC TILT MOVEMENT

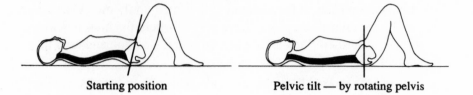

Starting position   Pelvic tilt — by rotating pelvis

The pelvic tilt is a good warm-up before you try the Back Power exercises. Most important, however, remember to adopt the pelvic tilt position *as you exercise.*

Getting Started: Ten Steps to Motivation

1) *Don't underestimate your problem.* "I'm okay, my back doesn't hurt now." "I'm fit enough. My job keeps me fit."

    When they aren't hurting, most people deny they have a back problem. That's why they may miss a golden opportunity to minimize future problems in *the easiest situation: when the back is pain-free.*

2) *Don't exaggerate your problem.* "I've had surgery on my back." "I've got arthritis." "My back is too weak for exercise."

    One irony of life is that, often, those of us who need help the most are the least likely to seek it. In general, the worse your back problem, the more you need back reconditioning exercises.

3) *Don't wait. Do it now.* "I know what to do — I'll just wait till my back hurts."

    Disease is reality. Health is taken for granted. To wait for your stroke or heart attack is to fail in management of your high blood pressure. Back pain is another failure in managing a problem. Good health is a commodity to be prized, to be valued, and to be worked for now!

4) *Don't overreach your capacity.* "I did my exercises and started to get pain. Exercise is not for me."

Some people are so eager to improve that they exercise with great vigor and intensity to the extent that pain results, and then discouragement is inevitable. The *"no pain means gain"* philosophy must be adopted for success.

5) *Don't fix blame. Fix the problem.* "My job . . . my chair . . . my shoes . . . cause my back problem."

Many people focus on external causes for their problem, and often these factors are beyond their control, leading to endless complaints and frustration. Make sure your own house is in order and that you keep your back fitness at the best level you can.

6) *Don't underestimate the Back Power program.* "Exercises are boring." "These exercises are too dull, too simple."

Back Power exercises have been designed after years of clinical experience with thousands of patients. These exercises were chosen *because they're simple* and hard to mess up. If they occasionally seem boring, so are brushing and flossing your teeth — but they're important to health management too.

7) *Be specific.* Commit yourself to a specific *time and place* for your daily exercises.

Make sure you know your *initial score* on the Back Power tests. *Track your progress.* Retest yourself weekly and record your results as you progress. If you are not improving, find out why: wrong exercise? wrong application?

8) *Affirm your goal.* "I will spend five minutes daily on Back Power exercise."

A positive affirmation is a very strong tool to ensure your commitment and consistency.

9) *Seek support — communicate your commitment.*

Express to your spouse or a friend your commitment to Back Power. Ask him or her to test you each week and encourage your partner to join you in the Back Power program.

10) *Dedicate yourself to solving your problem.* "I'm going to give it all I've got . . . to be the best I can possibly be."

The Back Power Exercises

Sling Stretch

How It Helps You
This exercise improves the length (flexibility) of your sling muscles.

How To Do It
1. Lie on your back, legs straight out.
2. Bring one knee toward your chest while the other leg remains straight out.
3. As you bring your knee toward your chest, you will feel increasing tension until you reach a "wall" where no further movement is possible; you may feel slight discomfort. *Stop*.
   - Loosen the knee off a little, and hold this position. Breathe in slowly and deeply.
   - Breathe out slowly until your lungs are empty. Relax.
   - Pause. Take up muscle slack by bringing your knee closer to your chest until you feel a new "wall."

FIG. 7.4   **SLING STRETCH**

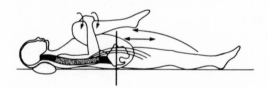

Repeat the Sling Stretch 3-5 times, then stretch your other sling muscle in your other leg.

Cautions
- Do not bounce.
- *No pain allowed* — only a gentle tension.
- Although breathing relaxes and stretches your muscles, *never force your limbs into a position*.
- If you feel pain in your sacroiliac joint, read chapter 6 and seek professional guidance.

Mad Cat

How It Helps You
This exercise stretches tight back muscles.

How To Do It
1. Get on all fours, on your hands and knees.
2. Try the three mad cat positions without attention to your breathing:
   - Neutral "level back" position.
   - Arch your back upward into a "dome" position, then back to the neutral level position.
   - Arch your back downward in a "suspension bridge" position, then back to neutral level position.
3. Now combine the three positions with deep breathing:
   - Neutral "level back" position: breathe in deeply.
   - Breathe out slowly as you assume the upward-arched "dome" position. Relax and stretch upward. Breathe in as you resume the level position.
   - Breathe out slowly as you assume the downward "suspension bridge" position. Relax and stretch downward. Resume neutral level position.

FIG. 7.5   **MAD CAT**

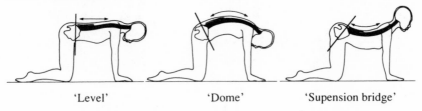

'Level'   'Dome'   'Supension bridge'

Repeat the Mad Cat 3-5 times.

Cautions
- Work gently.
- Breathe slowly and gently.
- Don't overstretch to the point of pain.

Side Stretch

How It Helps You
This exercise stretches tight lateral muscles.

How To Do It
1. Stand on both feet and clasp both hands on top of your head.

2. Bend sideways and slightly forward until you feel slight tightness in your lateral muscles. Hold this position.
   - Breathe in deeply.
   - Now breathe out deeply and feel the lateral muscles stretch as you get to the end of your breath.
   - Pause and relax. Take up slack in the muscles by bending further sideways and slightly forward.

FIG. 7.6   SIDE STRETCH

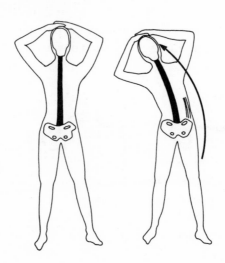

Repeat the Side Stretch 3-5 times.

Cautions
- Keep your hip bones square. Don't bend so far that your hip bones move sideways.
- Don't bounce or jerk.
- Breathe out completely before you stretch.

Sit-Down (and Curl)

How It Helps You

This is the first of Back Power's two power-strength exercises. Its purpose is to tighten long, out-of-shape stomach muscles.

How To Do It

1. Sit on the floor with both knees bent at a 45° angle and arms extended in front of you.

2. Slowly curl your trunk down to the floor, to a count of 7. Hold the pelvic tilt throughout.

FIG. 7.7 **SIT DOWN/CURL**

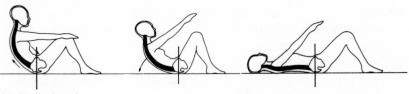

Sit-Down (easy)

3. Now, get back up to the sitting position, using arms to balance.

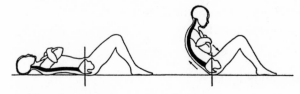

Sit-Down (moderate)

4. If this exercise is too easy, put your arms across your chest; to make it even harder, place your arms on the side of your head, slowly curl down, and sit back up again.

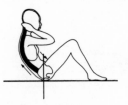

Sit-Down (difficult)

5. If this exercise is too hard, just try the *Curl*:
   - Lie on the floor, knees bent, arms extended in front of you.
   - Assume the pelvic tilt.
   - Slowly raise your body, curling yourself toward your knees. Hold to a count of 7 and return to starting position.

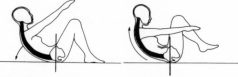

The Curl

Repeat the Sit-Down or Curl 5-10 times slowly.

Cautions
- Be comfortable. Don't progress to a harder level until you're strong enough.
- Sit back *slowly* for the best results.
- If you can't sit up easily, use your elbows to help you get up again.

Lateral Lift

How It Helps You
The Lateral Lift is Back Power's second power-strength exercise. Its purpose is to strengthen lateral muscles.

How To Do It
1. Lie on your side, legs straight out.
2. Cushion your head with one hand; use the other hand to support your body in a straight position on your side (think of the second hand as a post in a tripod).
3. Now raise both legs off the ground (2-4 inches). Hold this position.
4. Slowly raise and lower the upper leg in a scissorlike action.

FIG. 7.8 **LATERAL LIFT**

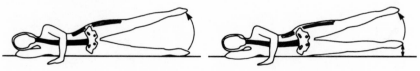

Repeat the Lateral Lift 5-10 times, then exercise the other side.

Cautions
- The higher you raise the lower leg, the harder the exercise.
- The easiest lateral lift position is with the lower leg on the ground.
- Keep your body perfectly straight for best results.
- To exercise your hip muscles, repeat the same exercise but tilt your body forward 15°. Feel the hip muscles work!

The Muscle Maintenance Program

The Muscle Maintenance program is suitable for people who received excellent scores on the Back Power tests. If your score was poorer than that, start on Muscle Maintenance once you have progressed through the Back Power exercise program (about six weeks). Muscle Maintenance serves as an excellent start to each day and as a warm-up routine before sports and other activity.

To the five Back Power exercises that you'll now be performing with ease, we add five new stretch-relaxation exercises and one power strength exercise.

Shoulder Stretch-Relaxation

How It Helps You
This exercise improves shoulder flexibility.

FIG. 7.9 SHOULDER STRETCH-RELAXATION

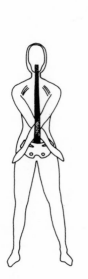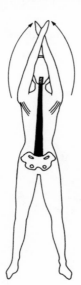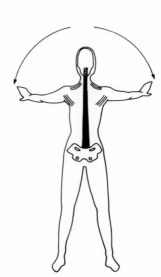

How To Do It

1. Let your arms dangle at your sides.
2. As you breathe in deeply, slowly raise your arms over your head, crossing your arms in front of you.
3. Now stretch your arms backward and into a circular motion as you slowly breathe out.
4. Repeat the process, stretching your arms backward as much as possible and enlarging the circles as you proceed.

Repeat the movement 3-5 times.

Groin Stretch-Relaxation

How It Helps You

This exercise improves groin flexibility.

How To Do It

1. Sit on the floor with knees bent to a 45° angle, heels together and 6 inches from your buttocks.
2. Push your knees outward with your elbows.
3. Bend your head downward toward your feet until you're stopped by muscle tightness.
4. Hold this position and breathe in deeply. Feel the relaxation response as you breathe in.
5. Breathe out slowly and pause at the end of your breath.
6. Now gently take up the slack by pushing both knees downward and your head toward your feet.

FIG. 7.10 **GROIN STRETCH-RELAXATION**

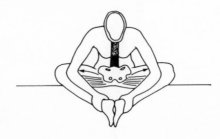

Repeat the movement 3-5 times.

Hamstring Stretch-Relaxation

How It Helps You
This exercise improves hamstring flexibility.

How To Do It
1. Sit with one leg bent, the sole of your foot near the knee of the straight leg.
2. Gently curl upper body toward the knee of the straight leg, and reach forward with your hands. Stop when you feel tension in your back or leg, but before the point of pain. Hold.
3. Breathe out slowly and deeply. Pause at the end of your breath. Feel the muscle relax.
4. Now gently take up the slack by bending your head further toward your knee.

FIG. 7.11 **HAMSTRING STRETCH-RELAXATION**

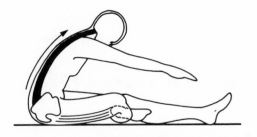

Repeat the movement 3-5 times, then stretch the other side.

Calf Stretch-Relaxation

How It Helps You
This exercise improves calf flexibility.

How To Do It
1. Stand with both feet on the floor, one in front of the other, and hands on your hips.
2. Bend your front leg to stretch the rear leg's calf muscle, keeping your rear foot flat on the floor and your rear leg straight.

3. When you feel tension in your calf muscle, stop and hold the position.
4. Now breathe out slowly and deeply. Feel the relaxation response.
5. Take up the slack in the muscle.

FIG. 7.12 CALF STRETCH-RELAXATION

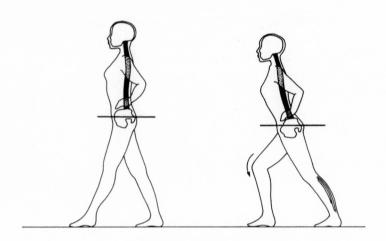

Repeat the movement 3-5 times, then stretch the other calf muscle.

Quadricep (Thigh) Stretch-Relaxation

How It Helps You
This exercise improves quad flexibility.

How To Do It
1. Stand on both feet with one shoulder against a wall to steady yourself.
2. Bring the heel of your outer foot toward your buttock. Hold the pelvic tilt position.
3. When you feel tightness in the thigh muscle, stop and hold the position.
4. Now breathe out slowly and deeply.
5. Take up the slack in the thigh muscle.

FIG. 7.13 QUADRICEP (THIGH) STRETCH-RELAXATION

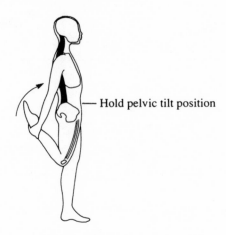

— Hold pelvic tilt position

Repeat the movement 3-5 times, then stretch the other leg.

Caution
• Do not arch your back.

The Power-Strength Push-Up

How It Helps You
This exercise provides shoulder and trunk muscle maintenance.

How To Do It

Easy
1. Get on all fours (as in the Mad Cat exercise), but let your knees touch the ground.
2. Move your hands forward a short distance.
3. Keeping your body perfectly straight, bend your elbows to lower your body and straighten them to raise your body from the floor.

Hard
1. Lie on your stomach, legs straight out and both hands on the floor under your shoulders.
2. Push up and down.

FIG. 7.14   THE POWER-STRENGTH PUSH-UP

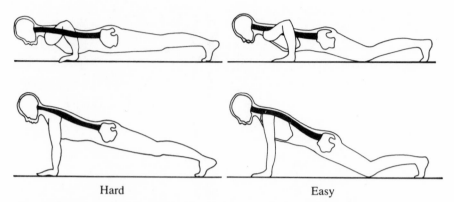

Hard   Easy

For both types of Push-Up, repeat the movement 5-10 times.

Muscle Maintenance for Life

Most people are surprised how easy these exercises are and how little time they take: about 10 minutes a day. But they are effective because they complement our daily activities and make up for deficiencies in our everyday life. They were designed to create balance of length and power of muscles.

Finally, they should be done daily, at the same time and in the same place. For maximum benefit they must be incorporated into your life, just as brushing your teeth and combing your hair are. Muscle maintenance is a life-skill.

In Review: Rules To Remember for Successful Exercise

Before we end this chapter, let's sum up the rules of the Back Power and Muscle Maintenance exercises.

1) If you're getting a lot of pain, you'll have no gain. Back Power is the no pain way to gain.

2) Remember the progressive overload principle. This simply means that you must push yourself a little bit in order to make progress. Start slowly, but be prepared to add to the difficulty or repetition of your exercises.

3) Pace yourself and stay within your personal limits. Don't try to become a superman or wonder woman in a week.

4) Remember to be comfortable. This has to be fun. Don't strain yourself. A little bit of discomfort may be okay at first, but there should not be a lot of pain.

5) Never forget the breathing. Gentle, relaxed breathing is the secret, especially for stretch-relaxation exercise.

6) Whenever possible, incorporate the pelvic tilt position into your exercises.

BACK POWER'S PROGRAMS FOR PREVENTION AND DISABILITY MANAGEMENT

8

Prevention:
The Name of the Game

This poem, recently reproduced in a medical journal, speaks volumes about the subject of this final chapter:

'twas a dangerous cliff, as they freely confessed,
    Though to walk near its crest was so pleasant;
But over its terrible edge there had slipped
    A duke and full many a peasant.
The people said something would have to be done,
    But their projects did not at all tally.
Some said, "Put a fence 'round the edge of the cliff,"
    Some, "An ambulance down in the valley."

The lament of the crowd was profound and was loud,
    As their hearts overflowed with their pity;
But the cry for the ambulance carried the day
    As it spread through the neighboring city.
A collection was made, to accumulate aid,
    And the dwellers in highway and alley
Gave dollars or cents — not to furnish a fence —
    But an ambulance down in the valley.

"For the cliff is all right if you're careful," they said;
    "And if folks ever slip and are dropping,
It isn't the slipping that hurts them so much
    As the shock down below — when they're stopping."
So for years (we have heard), as these mishaps occurred
    Quick forth would the rescuers sally,

125

To pick up the victims who fell from the cliff
　　With the ambulance down in the valley.

Said one, to his plea, "It's a marvel to me
　　That you'd give so much greater attention
To repairing results than to curing the cause;
　　You had much better aim at prevention.
For the mischief, of course, should be stopped at its source,
　　Come, neighbors and friends, let us rally
It is far better sense to rely on a fence
　　Than an ambulance down in the valley."

"He is wrong in his head," the majority said;
　　"He would end all our earnest endeavor,
He's a man who would shirk this responsible work,
　　But we will support it forever.
Aren't we picking up all, just as fast as they fall,
　　And giving them care liberally?
A superfluous fence is of no consequence,
　　If the ambulance works in the valley."

The story looks queer as we've written it here,
　　But things oft occur that are stranger.
More humane, we assert, than to succor the hurt,
　　Is the plan of removing the danger.
The best possible course is to safeguard the source
　　Attend to things rationally.
Yes, build up the fence and let us dispense
　　With the ambulance down in the valley.

A Champion of Prevention

Ralph Nader became a household name in the 1960s. This tough, young rabble-rousing lawyer would earn himself the nickname "the scourge of corporate morality," and it was well-deserved. Nader and his raiders were in the vanguard of a new movement for consumers' rights. In their concern and demands for better, safer automobile design, they would confront mighty manufacturers — and win the battle.

Whatever one's opinion of Nader and his methods, the fact remains that he achieved his goal. Cars are safer than ever before.

But no matter how safe the car, no matter how safe the highway, the other important variable is the most critical of all: the driver. Automobile safety is the result of a complex set of interactions between car and driver. Identifying and reducing risks in the car and driving environment must be coupled with reducing risks in the driver. But how do we approach the challenge?

On a global level, posters, ad campaigns, and TV jingles all promote safe driving habits. This is primary prevention: broadcasting the safe-driving message *before* the accident.

Then, we *target* specialized groups that are designated "high risk" drivers — young males in particular. Warnings against drinking and driving are widespread. Incentives are offered in the form of reduction in insurance costs when professional driving education is undertaken. This targeting effort is *secondary prevention.*

Tertiary prevention involves targeting chronically poor/dangerous drivers with intensive efforts to improve performance. Many states, for example, demand satisfactory completion of an interim safe-driving course if problem drivers are to retain their licenses.

Prevention of Low Back Problems

In a similar way, prevention of low back problems must include identification and reduction of risk in the job, the environment, the workplace, and the person. We know that injury, specifically, results from a mismatch between the demands of

risk in the job   &   risk in the person

▲

— a mismatch between a task and an individual's capability and strength.

In industry, there is a constant campaign to identify and reduce risk in the workplace by designing safer tasks, safer tools, and a safer environment. Policies implement better job training and protective equipment where required. Where it is used in industry, the Back Power initiative complements these efforts in reducing personal risk.

The Back Power program helps *all* back pain sufferers recover faster and better. But true primary prevention (*before* a bout of back pain or an injury) and secondary prevention (reconditioning a weak

back after a bout of pain or injury) is always a tough sell. The reason
is best summed up in this little proverb, sometimes called Imrie's
Law:

> **People's interest in and concern about their backs varies inversely with**
> **the length of time since they last suffered pain.**

In fairness, a variation of this law was known in the 16th century:

> **God and the Doctor, we alike adore**
> **But only when in danger, not before.**
> **The danger over, both are alike requited.**
> **God is forgotten, and the Doctor slighted.**
>
> — John Owen (1560-1622)

In other words, our perspective changes when we're not feeling *pain!*

A Sense of Perspective

Have you ever tried the nine-dot puzzle? It looks like this:

●   ●   ●

●   ●   ●

●   ●   ●

To solve the puzzle, you must join all nine dots by drawing only *four*
straight lines, never taking your pencil from the paper. (The solution
appears at end of this chapter.)

Most people have difficulty with this puzzle because their view
of it — their perspective — is restricted by the space confined by
the dots. When you look at the solution, you'll realize that the puzzle can be solved *only* by taking an unconventional and unrestricted
approach to the problem. That means looking at those dots from a
broader perspective.

In a similar way, the conventional perspective on backs and back
problems keeps us from really getting to the root of these problems
and managing them effectively.

Our Back Questionnaire

When we first interview a patient, we always ask these questions:

1) Have you ever had a back problem?
2) Do you have a problem now?
3) What caused your problem?
4) What do you do to prevent recurrence of the problem?

In this questionnaire, we emphasize the word *problem* rather than *pain*, yet people always answer the first two questions with a *pain* reference, a *pain* focus, a *pain perspective*. For example:

"Yes, doctor, I had a problem two years ago. But I'm fine now. I don't have any *pain*."

"Oh, yes. I had some *pain* about five years ago but I'm okay just now. My back may be a little weak — I'm not sure about that. But I'm feeling fine. I don't get any *pain*."

"Yes, I've had some *pain*. And I've still got a bit of a problem. When I get up in the morning, I feel stiff."

"Yes. I had a problem that started five years ago and I still get *pain* every day. This *pain*'s killing me. I've still got a problem all right!"

These answers to the two questions reflect how people think about back problems: they always equate a back problem with back pain.

A New Perspective

In this book, we present a program for measuring back health or function. We provide a tool that people can use
- to define a back problem not only when they have pain but also before they ever feel pain;
- to identify weak back dysfunction; or
- after having had pain, to ascertain whether there is a burden of injury — a susceptibility to future back trouble.

This new perspective is important because it stresses prevention and management. Our goal is to make people look at their backs and back problems in a new way. What follows is a useful analogy.

Relationship between Health and Disease

High Blood Pressure — A Painless Example

We all know that high blood pressure over many years puts added strains on the heart, which has to pump harder against the higher head of pressure, and on the blood vessels, where it accelerates degeneration and aging. The consequences of high blood pressure are a greater risk of heart disease, heart attack, and stroke. And we know that people have a problem when they experience the chest pain of a heart attack or the weakness of a stroke.

With high blood pressure, however, neither the public nor our health professionals wait for such calamities to occur before treating the problem. The condition is easily identified with the band and meter device called a *sphygmomanometer*. Hypertension (high blood pressure) is an asymptomatic or *unhurting* problem that is usually detected long before the onset of any serious consequences. It is a problem that can be managed by the individual so that no irreversible changes in the heart and blood vessels need ever occur. Aggressive care of the high blood pressure problem before the catastrophe is so routine that, in the health professions, we almost consider it a failure of management if someone suffers a heart attack or a stroke!

People have a clear understanding that high blood pressure is a problem even though *it is a painless condition*. From the individual's point of view, then, there is seldom resistance to the need to alter the diet, take any necessary medication, and watch activity levels so as to lower the blood pressure.

This is a good example of the relationship between health and disease. Let's stress once again that health is *not* just the absence of disease, heart attack, or stroke — or the feeling that "everything is okay." Health must be defined in terms of optimal function when compared with a health standard. In our example, high blood pressure is most certainly not optimal function.

Management and Maintenance

Oral hygiene offers another good example to illustrate health management and disease treatment. After your dentist has treated any cavities or gum problems you may have, he or she is unlikely to say, "Come back if you have pain." Good dentists ensure that their patients are well-versed in maintenance of oral hygiene through daily brushing and flossing. Good oral health is a joint concern: the best from the treating professional and the individual's own best efforts. A pain in the tooth is a failure in management of the system.

You and Your Back

O ur goal is to make people realize that back pain is the failure in management of back health. Back pain is not the start of a problem, it is the end result. It represents the progressive breakdown of a mechanical system. It is the result of excessive risks and decreasing back health over a period of time.

If you've had back pain and it has gone away, don't imagine that your back is "healthy now" and that you can resume all previous activities. Rather, you must be aware that back pain always leaves a back weakened and susceptible to the next problem.

How Back Problems Begin

W hen asked the third question on our *Back Questionnaire, what caused your back problem?* most people tell us what they were doing when the pain occurred:

"I was lifting the baby out of the crib."

"I was getting the beer out of the back of the car."

"I was shoveling snow."

"I slipped and fell."

"I was lifting something heavy at work."

A surprisingly large number of people can't account for the specific cause of the pain. They'll say something like:

"I got out of bed in the morning and had this pain. It got worse as the day went on. At one point, I bent over to fix my shoelaces and I couldn't straighten up."

Sometimes people even attribute back pain to something they did in the recent past. For example: "I cut the lawn three days ago and I'm feeling bad today."

In all this, the key point is that people almost invariably look *externally* for the cause of their pain — at problems or risk in their job or their immediate environment. Whether they associate their back pain with a specific event, whether they attribute it to an event in the recent past, or whether they can't pinpoint an exact event, the tendency is for people to have a one-dimensional perspective when they ascribe the cause of their pain.

What interests us greatly is that so many activities that people attribute their back pain to are activities of daily function — things done day in and day out, year in and year out: lifting the baby; getting the beer out of the trunk; cutting grass; shoveling snow. None of these activities is new or unusual for the people concerned. At the same time, it is relatively uncommon for us to see people who are suffering back injury because of car accidents, a fall from a great height, or a football mishap — in short, any bad accidents that have overwhelmed the ability of the body to cope.

If, however, our perspective on the cause of back problems is so one-dimensional, then our solution will be to alter our activities: we'll stop shoveling snow, cutting the grass, lifting the baby. But does that *really* make sense? We believe — and that should be apparent by now — that a broader, multidimensional perspective must be adopted when considering back problems.

The Risk Factor

That said, we must also point out that there are, of course, inherent risks in a job, an activity, or the environment. A great deal of research has been done over the years to define these risks. We now know that there are basically six specific risks:

1) The heavier the load, the greater the risk to the back.
2) If a twisting movement is involved in lifting a heavy load, abnormal stress will be placed on the back.
3) Jobs with a vibration element — like driving a truck or other heavy vehicle — seem to predispose individuals to back problems.
4) Conversely, jobs that do not have a lot of movement in them — like driving a car or sitting at a work station for prolonged periods — have the same predisposition.
5) Jobs that have abnormal postures which create excessive muscular action or static loading also carry a risk factor.
6) Situations where a weight shifts suddenly while being lifted can also create problems (an ambulance attendant's work, for example).

Most of the effort devoted to studies of back problems has looked at modifying one or more of these six risk factors, particularly in the work environment. We believe, however, that it is also essential to look at the other component in question: the person.

Back Power and the Individual

T he Back Power program has been developed to help individuals define risks in *themselves* — risks of diminished back strength and flexibility that may occur before a back problem develops and that certainly occur as a direct result of a mechanical back problem once it exists.

Let's use the seesaw analogy again:

demands of the task   &   back fitness (capability) of the person

▲

In this perspective, we can see how back problems emerge as a mismatch between these two risk factors: *external tasks* and *personal capability*. We can say that high risk jobs require strong individuals; conversely, excessive risk and weakness in the individual produce an inability to function even in the normal activities of daily living.

Epidemiology: Two Studies for Prevention

E pidemiology is the study of the distribution of a disease in a given group of people. It is an extremely useful research method because it often gives us clues about major preventive or management processes for a disease.

For example, one of the major epidemiological studies that linked heart disease to a sedentary life-style focused on the bus drivers and bus conductors of London's Transport Commission. Here were individuals working in the same environment over many years. The difference, however, was that the driver was sitting down all day (sedentary, though under high stress and pressure), but the conductor was walking — climbing up and down stairs in the double-decker buses or standing to collect the passengers' fares.

The research showed that heart disease and heart attacks were much more frequent in the sedentary bus drivers than in the active conductors who worked in the same environment. This classic study was one of many which proved that heart disease and inactivity are linked and ultimately led to today's fitness boom.

Other important epidemiological evidence is that of the association between lung cancer and smoking. This link was seen in men for many years, though many people, including some professionals, insisted that it was unproven.

Recently, lung cancer has overtaken breast cancer as the major type of the disease in women, a fact almost totally attributed to the increase in smoking among women after the second World War and the consequences seen 20 to 30 years later.

These are two examples of epidemiological studies; there are countless others.

Recurrence of Back Problems

Our fourth and final *Back Questionnaire* question is, *what do you do to prevent recurrence of the problem?* Of all the replies, three general responses predominate.

The first type of response is, "I have to live with it. There's nothing that can be done about my pain." Or sometimes, more sadly, "I have to live with the pain until it's bad enough to have surgery."

The people in this group are resigned to the notions that their pain will continue and probably worsen in the future, and that they themselves have very little input or control over the problem. They may feel rejected by health professionals, whom, they perceive as not really understanding the magnitude or intensity of their pain, or whom they may regard as callous and insensitive to their needs. There are patients who have told us that their doctor would not perform surgery because "they don't believe I'm bad enough yet."

The second common response is a behavioral one. Respondents in this group go out of their way to avoid any risks in their job or environment that are likely to induce or worsen their back pain. They avoid all sports, most household activities, and relevant job activities. They may even change jobs. Here we see a loss of control over one's life and, even more important, a loss of *quality* in one's life.

The final response is usually active in a passive way. This third group includes people who take medication to lessen their back pain or go for treatments when their pain worsens. In order to carry on, people in this group may be on maintenance/fitness programs or maintenance/care programs with physiotherapists or chiropractors.

What all these people have in common is knowledge that their back is weak but *lack* of knowledge about what they can do to manage the problem. They have no sense of standards or measurements that they can apply to determine their health deficiency or dysfunctional problems. And they are unaware of the constructive steps they can take to turn their problem around. These people are living in pain, their lives are pain-centered, and their behavior is determined by pain. Indeed, pain has become their "malevolent dictator," decreeing what they can and cannot do.

The Back Power program described in this book can help to change all that. The critical ingredient is *you*.

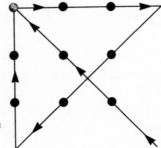

Solution to the nine-dot puzzle
(p. 128)

9

Managing the Disability Process

This was no ordinary man. This young, handsome athlete had just completed a 25,000-mile round-the-world journey — one in which he'd battled the heat of the Great Victoria Desert in Australia, blinding dust storms in China, the fatigue of a tough journey through the Alps, and the wearying distances of the long, long road called the Trans-Canada Highway — all 4,888 miles of it.

Fourteen years before, on a rainy, windy mountain road, the truck in which this young man — then 15 years old — was riding had skidded out of control on the slick pavement, flipping over in a dreadful accident that left him paralyzed from the waist down.

The young man's name is Rick Hansen. His journey was called the Marathon of Hope. During 1986-87, Hansen traveled those 25,000 miles in his wheelchair. His goals were two: first, to prove that people with disabilities can achieve "the impossible"; second, to raise funds for research on spinal cord injuries.

"What counts," says Hansen, "is not the disability but the ability." Rick Hansen, a paraplegic, behaved as if he had no disability. His attitude speaks for itself.

Coming to Terms with Disability

Rick Hansen, like the victim of any serious accident who is left with significant organic pathology, had to live through many contrasting phases of attitude before coming to terms with disability.

At first, these people react with *denial*: "I *can't* be that bad. I'm sure I'll get better."

Then *rationalization*: "It could have been worse. At least I'm *alive*."

Then *anguish*: "I'm finished. What am I going to do? I'll never be the same again."

Then *determination*: The search for hope — a cure — a miracle. Waiting in countless waiting rooms, consulting any number of gurus for an answer; tests and more tests, hopes and expectations raised only to be dashed. Seeking that elusive diagnosis, prognosis, *cure*.

But when no such answer is found, a sense of despair sets in as grief. The idea of a changed life, changed plans, and lack of control leads to a loss of self-esteem — to feelings of worthlessness.

Now the primitive instinct of "fight or flight" surges to the surface. Flight — giving up — might be the path to the sheltered workshop. Fight means regaining control.

Beginning the Fight

Determination to overcome requires a series of steps for success:

1) Evolve a plan. This gives a sense of direction and, down the road, a *goal*.

2) Make sure the plan is realistic. Always remember to *accept what you can't change and change what you can*. It is at this point that realistic acceptance replaces the free-floating search for the elusive cure.

3) Make *hope* your watchword — but base it on achievable goals.

4) Seek and accept support — from family, friends, health professionals, the community.

As you regain self-esteem and start to become interdependent — relying much more on that support from family, friends, and others — you start on the road to renewed independence. It's time to rely on praise instead of pity. Time to try behaving like Rick Hansen, as if you were *fully functional*.

When Back Pain Disables

Human existence is defined by two essential activities: *I think*; *I do*. With the exception of the intellect, our bodies are organized for movement: to work, to nurture, to eat, to play — to *function*, in short.

It is not surprising, then, that no group of disorders is so common and disturbing as those manifested by pain in general and spinal pain in particular. Despite the scientific methods of investigation and advanced therapeutic techniques, solutions to the problem back are still wanting.

Inherent in all human beings is a feeling of immortality, which is threatened only in times of vulnerability: sickness, old age, loss. Illness also creates a sense of insecurity.

In most cases of illness we recover, though in some we remain with residual chronic problems. Both recovery and chronic situations are usually accepted, eventually. A much more difficult situation exists, however, when an individual feels ill and disabled but no cause or diagnosis can be found: there is no specific treatment and no prognosis — no certainty of what will happen in the future.

Uncertainty is a debilitating state in itself and the cornerstone of the disability process.

Rick Hansen and others like him who have successfully coped with chronic disease and injury are ultimately liberated by an acceptance of reality — bad though it is — and reacting positively to the new challenges facing them.

Doctor! Doctor! Fix My Back!

The perceptions of patients and health professionals alike are based on a mechanistic view of the universe and the expectation of a "quick fix," a miracle cure. In our modern age, these expectations sometimes even come true. Actions are based on the belief that back pain is caused by a physical pathological condition:

Cause   →   Effect
(injury; structural problem)   (back pain)

As we've seen, this scientific method of dealing with disease has been proven effective over the years because, in many conditions, *it works*. For the vast majority of back pain sufferers, however, it does not work. For the vast majority of back pain, the treatment is palliative and passive: rest, heat, and analgesics. And that works. The back pain usually disappears. Studies show that:

45% of back pain disappears in 1 week
80% of back pain disappears in 4 weeks
90% of back pain disappears in 8 weeks

The usual natural history of back pain is disappearance of the symptom within two months, regardless of the treatment given! At the same time, however, the rule of back problems is *recurrence*. Once painful or injured, a back usually becomes a problem again and again — each bout more severe than the last.

THE PROGRESSION OF LOW BACK PAIN

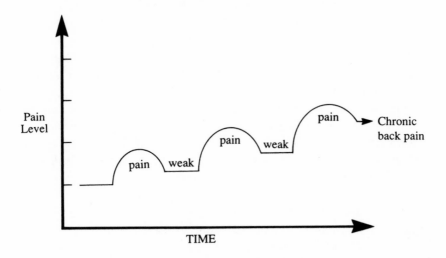

In the early stages, the conditioned response of injury → rest (passivity) = success (relief from pain) reinforces the patient's view of the world that injury causes a mechanical failure made better by rest. This view supports the "quick fix" mentality that persists in many patients later in the disease process, when conservative measures no longer successfully deal with pain.

The *disability process* begins when the pain becomes chronic but is not associated with a correctable defect and does not respond to palliative measures. Still, the mechanistic view that was so successful previously is championed by way of a search for a better test, a better practitioner, a better pill, or a more potent treatment. This sequence usually becomes one of raised expectations and dashed hopes. It's not hard to see how the physical problems are soon overshadowed by emotional reactions in the patient — uncertainty, anger, and finally despair.

Responses to Low Back Disability

The key word we use to describe many chronic low back disabilities is "inappropriate."

We talk about inappropriate disability — *too much* disability compared with the objective organic abnormalities.

We refer to inappropriate use of medication — in amount, combinations, and potency. Attempts to reduce medication may generate anger in the patient and guilt in the doctor: "It's my pain. You don't believe how bad it is. Help me be comfortable."

We describe inappropriate symptoms, including many that are hard to measure (with otherwise normal findings): headache, fatigue, insomnia, neck ache — all in spite of rest.

Inappropriate emotions run the gamut: depression or discouragement, focused mainly on the inability to find out what is wrong and thus be able to do something about it; anger at the treating professional who is often challenged by the patient to diagnose the problem and relieve the suffering; anger at supervisors or fellow employees who may be perceived to have caused the problem or who don't believe its severity; anger at insuring agencies for questioning the legitimacy of payments or for delaying payments; passivity — taking the utmost care to rest and avoid further injury; hopelessness — a feeling of loss of personal control and power.

And finally we refer to inappropriate behavior, supported and "proven" by significant alterations in life-style (invalidism, being on medication, venturing forth only for treatments or to obtain prescriptions).

The inappropriate response of the sufferer does not occur in a vacuum but develops in the wider context of work, home, and community. Thus the reaction of others *to* the disabled person is just as important in the development of the disability process as is the subjective reaction *in* that person.

A family's, spouse's, friend's initial reaction to back disability is concern, sympathy, support, and help. As the months go by with no new answers, as housework and bills pile up, as basic needs are not satisfied and the future becomes uncertain, concern turns first to neutrality and then to downright indifference — even hostility and rejection. Family and friends at first are enablers — supporting the disability — but uncertainty can change that role.

As health professionals, our main goal in life is serving patients, healing the sick, easing suffering. No greater compliment can be paid than, "Doctor, thanks to you I feel great!" Sadly, chronic backs seldom produce such rewarding results, a fact that creates frustration in both patient and practitioner.

Costs of Low Back Disability

The importance of the relationship between the patient and the practitioner is run a close second by that between the patient and the insuring agency responsible for replacement income benefits. The physician is the source of help and cure; the insurer, the source of financial security.

Payment for sickness is usually automatic at first, but after a few months insuring agencies usually have a second look at disability cases and employers start to scrutinize the claim, which is now costing megadollars. This process only adds to the emotional distress of the patient: *anger*, because scrutiny appears equivalent to disbelief of the condition or its severity; *fear* that financial hardship is imminent. When a third-party assessment is called for, it is seen as a threat. For reasons of personal integrity, vindication, or financial security, the patient's effort then may be concentrated not on getting well but on proving the existence of the disability.

The combination of anger, fear, and frustration often leads the patient into the waiting arms of the legal profession. And at this point the disability process usually becomes firmly entrenched. More assessment, more tests, more opinions: directed *not* at elucidation of the problem and healing, *not* at altering dysfunction and mitigating loss, but again at *proving how sick* and disabled the individual is.

Many studies have indicated that the longer a person is disabled and dysfunctional, the *less* likely he or she is to return to an active, productive life, regardless of the amount of organic pathology. When behavior patterns of sickness and invalidism become firmly entrenched, they are extremely difficult to dislodge. Chronic pain is more than a sensory perception. It is a total disarrangement of a person's behavior and life-style.

Why Disability?

In chapter 2, we illustrated what goes on inside a person to produce a pain behavior response. The manifestations of this response are basically three: (1) some accept the pain and carry on with life; (2) others react in just the opposite way, determined to "rest up" so that the body can heal properly; and (3) still others begin a quest to find that elusive health professional who can diagnose and treat their pain.

The disability process is a complex behavioral response less dependent on the *disease* in the person than on the person's *reaction* to the disease. Managing the disability process is a challenge far removed from dealing with a broken leg or an appendix operation. In the following section we offer an approach for management.

A Recipe for Action

Having dealt with how the disability process becomes established, we now offer an approach for *managing* this process: a recipe for action. By way of introduction, this diagram will help demonstrate the factors at work.

FIG. 9.2 **THE DISABILITY PROCESS**

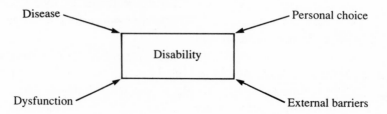

Four Factors

As shown in the diagram, we see that disability is a complex interaction of four factors: disease, dysfunction, personal choice, and external barriers.

Disease
Disease is an organic pathological condition. It means that something is wrong. Some change, such as a fracture or tumor, has taken place in the normal structure of the body. Disease is defined by specific symptoms, and it can be confirmed by specific tests that are reproduceable by different practitioners and lead to a specific diagnosis. Each diagnosis has specific therapies and a prognosis, or expected outcome. Disease may or may not produce *dysfunction*.

Dysfunction

Dysfunction is the loss of normal capability to do something. It means that a specific organ, joint, or group of joints — as in the low back — is not working as it was designed to work.

With reference to the low back, dysfunction can mean a loss of range of movement, a loss of muscular strength, a loss of muscle *balance*, or fixation or instability of the joints.

An important point to note is that just as disease does not necessarily cause dysfunction, dysfunction in turn is not necessarily the result of disease. Take the individual with asymptomatic narrowing of the blood vessels to the heart but no signs of dysfunction or pain. Contrast this potential heart attack victim with the unfit person who runs a mile for the first time in years and experiences tightness in the chest with extreme shortness of breath — but has no significant disease. In this way, we make the point that very little low back pain is related to identifiable organic pathologies. Pain indicates something wrong. Most people think the problem is because of disease when in fact it's because of dysfunction.

Disability itself is the sum total of attitudes, beliefs, and behaviors of an individual who is dysfunctional — whether or not as the result of disease. The approach to this disability may be *appropriate* to the condition (resting after a recent broken leg) or *inappropriate* (resting a stiff finger that really needs to be moved). Regardless, it has a strong component of our third factor: personal choice.

Personal Choice

If someone says, "My back pain *prevents* me" from doing this or that, what he or she may be expressing is an unwillingness to do this or that because the pain hurts too much, because there is fear of the consequences of the action, because of fear of what the pain means or because of some other reason. This personal choice may be based on a number of factors.

The belief system of the individual. If the individual believes that the pain is *harm* pain — that activity will be harmful — then such activity will be avoided. Someone who believes instead that activity will be *hurtful* but is *necessary* to improve the situation, will choose to become active in spite of the discomfort.

Consequences of the choice. If it is more desirable to remain sick and disabled than it is to become well, for example when there is potential for a large monetary settlement after an injury or accident, then the personal choice of disability can become the more attractive choice.

Willingness to alter life-style or behavior in order to mitigate loss and improve the situation. An individual can have a significant amount of disease in the low back and yet mitigate loss by improving function, mobility, and muscle strength. It is sometimes necessary to experience significant discomfort in order to ease the situation. Personal choice is clearly the most critical factor in the disability process, yet it is the part of the equation most often ignored.

External Barriers

Disability can sometimes be fostered in otherwise keen people by external barriers in the environment. For example, an individual in a wheelchair might be capable and prepared to do a certain job but unable to gain access to the premises because no ramp is available. *Other people* sometimes influence the status of the disability process — even with the best intentions in the world.

The Disability Perspective

Our diagram for viewing disability is extremely important not only to allow us to assess each situation from the same perspective but to help explain to our patients how they are, in fact, part of the solution. Each individual's choice and willingness to mitigate loss is an essential part of managing the disability process.

In concluding this chapter, we offer to the patient and the practitioner seven steps toward management of low back disability.

Seven Steps toward Managing Low Back Disability

Affirmation — Being Clear with the Patient

Affirmation means defining clearly whether or not significant organic disease is present. If none is found, the patient must be helped to a better understanding of the cause of his or her problem. A negative X-ray, for example, is a golden opportunity to reassure the patient and focus on that other vital part of the back — the muscles.

Whether or not the cause of low back disability is disease, a *crucial* first step is being clear with the patient. Misinformation or miscommunication can lead to extreme mental anguish or inappropriate behaviors, with the patient taking on *the attitudes of disability.*

Explanation — What Does Pain Mean?

As we've seen, it is most important that patients understand the difference between *harm* pain and *hurt* pain.

Harm pain indicates that something is physically wrong. After acute injury such as a fractured leg, the pain serves a *useful function*, telling us that activity/movement will cause problems, delaying healing. Acute pain is *harmful* and creates a positive behavioral response — rest, splint, or cast for a fracture — to *promote* health and healing.

Hurt pain — discomfort, soreness, stiffness — also indicates that something is wrong, but it dictates a different response. With hurt pain, activity/exercise is *usually* indicated. Hurt pain is often part of the *progressive overload principle* necessary to improve fitness. Hurt pain in ankylosing spondylitis or in the segmental instability of degenerative disc disease, for example, is part of the "hurt" sacrifice necessary for living; it cannot "harm" the patient.

Patients need guidance on the nature of their pain and the appropriate behavioral response. Many people with low back problems never experience significant pain but, failing to understand the distinction between *harm* and *hurt*, fear to do *anything* that might cause pain.

Definition — Function, Dysfunction

Understand the meanings of function and dysfunction and form a coherent treatment plan based on restoration of balance to muscles and movement to joints.

Transformation — Changing the Focus

Accept the structural changes, which are a reality and cannot be changed, and change the muscular and joint dysfunction. These key steps will change the focus from pain (hurt pain, harm pain) to movement, activity, and positive behaviors:

- Channel emotional energy to positive, healthy pursuits.
- Disassociate activity from pain.
- Move from passive to active control.
- Eliminate drugs where possible. Drugs can alter mood and feeling; they are not part of the solution and will usually only contribute to the disability process.

Dedication — Taking Control

"Am I willing to take control to be the best I can possibly be?" It may hurt, but it is up to the health professional to interpret hurt vs. harm.

Knowing, then, that you'll be monitored to ensure that you're not harmed or deteriorating, this step becomes a matter of *personal choice*.

Evaluation, Monitoring, and Coaching —
The Ongoing Relationship between Patient and Practitioner

The ongoing relationship between patient and practitioner now becomes one of management, not treatment; of support and coaching to better, healthier attitudes; of more effective fitness and exercise techniques while Mother Nature heals. Of course, the health professional is there to "help you up if you should fall down" in the future — if there is a recurrence of your spinal problem.

Prevention and Maintenance —
Managing the Disability Process

The pain may be gone, but you've made a commitment: to be the best you can possibly be; to carry on with exercise and fitness routines; and to manage the disability process. This brings us to Imrie's second law: *When the pain settles down, it's time to start managing your problem.*

MORE ABOUT BACK POWER

10

Case Histories

Back Power Tests: Review of Scoring	
Excellent	1
Good	2
Fair	3
Poor	4

A.   The Major Cause of Back Pain

CASE HISTORY #1: COMMON BACKACHE

NAME: Dave

AGE: 35

One of our patients, Dave, is 35 and works as a laborer. He has suffered several bouts of back pain in recent years. At the time of our first consultation he was pain-free, having recovered several months earlier from his most recent bout. Dave had become increasingly concerned about his capabilities and was eager to take the Back Power tests.

A big, well-muscled man, he was participating in a fair amount of sport, though he'd cut back his activities somewhat. Dave was quite sure he'd breeze through the tests with no trouble. But here is his score:

1) Sit-Up Test	4	(back flexibility)	
2) Leg Raise Test	1	(stomach strength)	
3) Sling Test (L, 3 / R, 1 ÷ 2)	2	(sling flexibility)	
4) Lateral Lift Test (L, 3/R, 1 ÷ 2)	2	(lateral flexibility & strength)	
Total	**9**	(a *fair* score)	

Dave's flexion and extension tests each scored 4, indicating a major loss of range of movement.

His scores surprised Dave, but he was puzzled by something else. The initial bout of severe back pain that had laid him up so badly occurred on his *left* side, where his sling and lateral muscles were clearly much weaker than those on the right. His next bout of pain, however, occurred on his *right* side: How come? We explained that the muscles on his right side had to work overtime to try to compensate for the weakness on the left. Dave had had some chiropractic treatment, which gave him a degree of relief when he had trouble. The unequal muscle balance had created mechanical stress in the low back, which was helped for a time with adjustment. Discomfort soon occurred, however, necessitating further therapy.

Back Power Program

We explained to Dave that he had large muscle bulk but poor flexibility. We demonstrated how lack of muscle length produces weakness and how work and exercise create muscle shortness (the state we call "musclebound"), which also creates weakness. Dave was intrigued. He knew all about strength exercise but considered stretching to be "sissy stuff."

We next explained to Dave that although all the Back Power exercises (chapter 7) were desirable, he must emphasize reconditioning in his specific areas of weakness, as follows:

Area of Weakness	Exercise
1) back flexibility	Mad Cat
2) stomach strength	Sit-Downs
3) sling flexibility	Sling Stretch (left)
4) lateral flexibility and strength	Side Stretch (left)
	Lateral Lift

Dave committed to a five-minute-a-day routine. In one week we retested him. These were his results:

1) Sit-Up Test	3
2) Leg Raise Test	1
3) Sling Test	1
4) Lateral Lift Test	1
Total	**6**

This time, Dave scored *2* on extension and *3* on flexion — the closest he'd been to his toes in years!

Dave not only saw the improvement in back test function but also *felt* different. He said he was now less tired at the end of his workday and had more energy for personal activities. He was amazed that with relatively little effort, he'd made such progress in so little time.

B.   Low Back Disease and the Back Power Program

CASE HISTORY #2: HERNIATED DISC
NAME: Frank
AGE: 53

Our patient, Frank, describes himself as a changed man. Before his injury, he'd always been active — a hard worker. One of his jobs was delivering heavy appliances; he had no difficulty hauling a washing machine from his truck and down a basement. Once happy-go-lucky, nothing seemed to bother him. Now, with constant discomfort, it doesn't take much to put a chip on his shoulder at work or at home. His present job, changed because of his back problems, is light survey work that does involve some walking — a good thing in his case — when he's able to work at all.

At 53, Frank says he often feels 90. At the time of our last appointment he had been off work with chronic back and leg pain for two months, and though he says his back is a little better, he still has to sit down to ease on his underpants and trousers. His wife has to help him with his shoes and socks — he can't bend over far enough to put them on.

Seven years ago, Frank injured his back in a bad fall. Though he had severe pain at the time of the accident, he could still move about quite normally. The next day, however, he had great difficulty moving at all. He had back and leg pain as well as stiffness.

Initially, he was advised that he had a "low back strain." He was prescribed painkillers and told to lie flat as much as possible until the pain began to ease. When there was little improvement, Frank sought therapy, but found it actually aggravated his pain to the point he was laid up again. Unable even to move without pain, Frank had to rely on his wife for everything — even helping him to the washroom.

After several weeks of desperation, doped on pills, struggling with therapy, resting all the time, he was referred to a specialist for neuro-orthopedic assessment. But the surgeon was available only for "emergency cases" — it would be six weeks before he could see Frank. That really upset Frank. His problem certainly felt like an emergency, and the shambles of his present life proved the point.

Six weeks passed like six years. When he finally saw the surgeon, indications of herniated disc meant that no further time was wasted in testing Frank further. CATscan followed by myelogram were conclusive: a herniated disc at the L5/S1 level. This disc was putting pressure on the nerve to his left leg, causing numbness in his foot, searing sciatic pain in his leg, and weakness of his ankle movement.

Frank was shocked to learn that herniated disc was first dealt with by "conservative care": heat, rest, and analgesics. He was to endure another six weeks of complete bed rest, but the problem progressed relentlessly. Surgery was the only hope. Finally! The problem was to be fixed.

For the first two years after his surgery, Frank had no recurrence of back pain or leg problems. Then came two painful experiences, when he could not bend over or sit with comfort. The pain was less severe than it had been previously, however, and didn't progress down his legs.

The following year, the problem recurred and Frank was off work for three or four weeks. The attacks of pain were more frequent and the leg pain returned. Frank would return to work for a time, only to be laid up again with his pain.

Now, his leg pain is present all the time unless he sits down. When he lies down, some positions are comfortable, some agonizing. His leg has been very numb lately. When his condition is at its worst, Frank can't drive. He describes a situation where he would have to lift his bad leg with his hand in order to place his foot on the brake.

Frank takes Tylenol 3, which gives some relief from his pain but causes other problems, constipation especially. Frank believes he has literally "tried everything" for his pain, but really to no avail. Convinced that surgery had helped him once, he finally came to believe that it could help him again. But a recent CATscan failed to show a surgical problem. Frank was dumbfounded. His hope vanished. No cure. Condemned to live with his pain.

Then a friend referred him to us for assessment. Could Back Power help?

Test Results and Back Power Program
When we tested Frank, we found a fairly typical picture of someone who has had chronic back pain as well as previous surgery.

On the Sit-Up test, he scored *4*. This grade indicated tremendous inflexibility in his back resulting from age and previous surgery.

The Straight Leg test was, surprisingly, his best score, at *2*, indicating fairly good stomach muscle tone.

The sling muscles scored a *4* on the right and a *3* on the left. Laterals were a *4* on the left and a *3* on the right. These scores had immediate meaning for Frank. He'd had major pain down his left leg although now it was in both legs, and he could see significant asymmetry between the two sides.

Frank's total score was *13*.

No more could be done for Frank surgically. But the fact that he had a high degree of dysfunction meant that if he was prepared to commit himself to an exercise routine, the indications for significant improvement were good.

We started Frank on Back Power exercises, stressing flexibility in particular: the Mad Cat, Sling Stretch, and Lateral Stretch at first; then, after a gradual increase in repetitions of these exercises, he expanded a few weeks later to Curl and Lateral Leg Lift.

After a few months, Frank's score improved to *7*. With constant effort, he'll be able to do better still. Most important, however, is that Frank now feels he can control his destiny. His back function is improving. He *feels* much better.

CASE HISTORY #3: ANKYLOSING SPONDYLITIS

NAME: Rob

AGE: 23

Rob, in the prime years of his life at 23, should have been full of vigor, happy and challenging life. But he sat in the consulting room looking downcast and pale, tired, depressed, and confused. His story was quite typical.

Four years before, the problem had started with stiffness in his low back on each side of his tail bone. It wasn't too bad at first, and Rob noticed that so long as he was moving about actively, the pain would go away. But it didn't *stay away*. In fact, it became progressively worse, to the extent that it began to affect Rob's work and his outlook.

When Rob went for assessment, little was found. His X-rays were normal. Pills provided good relief at first, but in time even these stopped working and the pain began spreading up his back.

On our first consultation, it was obvious that Rob's problem was not only physical but was having a profound effect on his mental outlook. His fiancée, who accompanied him, confirmed that Rob was a grouch.

Complete examination revealed nothing except a little stiffness on moving the back. X-rays were normal. So were blood tests for the presence of inflammatory arthritis. In a young man, however, the symptom of pain on waking did point to arthritis, even though we could not yet prove it. One specialist and a bone scan later, the diagnosis was confirmed: ankylosing spondylitis.

Anti-inflammatory medication helped the physical problem. Clearing up the uncertainty and being able to give Rob a prognosis started to lift his depression. Could anything else be done to manage Rob's condition?

Test Results and Back Power Program

Rob's pattern in the tests was quite typical for an individual with ankylosing spondylitis.

On the Sit-Up test he scored *4*, reflecting the severe degree of stiffness that had set in. All other results were quite good: *1* on the Straight Leg Raise, indicating strong stomach muscles; and *2* on each of the Sling tests, showing a degree of tightness from athletic pursuits in the not-too-distant past. Completing the picture was a score of *1* on the right and *2* on the left in the Lateral tests.

Rob's total score was 8.5, but almost half of that was on account of the stiffness in his back in the Sit-Up test.

Rob already had been given exercises, but our tests highlighted how deficient he was in the area of back flexibility. This pinpointing of his problem, as well as an awareness of the difference between *hurt* (discomfort) pain and *harm* pain, motivated Rob to redouble his efforts. He put special emphasis on the Mad Cat and other flexibility exercises for the back.

Rob's discomfort and stiffness would be with him for many years to come, but he was now determined to minimize them to the greatest extent possible.

CASE HISTORY #4: SPONDYLOLISTHESIS
NAME: Janet
AGE: 30

Janet, 30, usually ignored minor aches and pains and Mother Nature usually took good care of her. She prided herself on her good health and good fortune, her strong athletic body. But this pain was different.

This winter, she slipped on the ice on her walk. What a jab of pain! And it lingered.

Finally, Janet sought professional help. Examination and X-rays soon pointed to spondylolisthesis as the cause — an instability in the bones of Janet's low back.

The doctor explained that the defect had been present since birth, but the fall — even such a minor one — must have aggravated the condition. This explanation surprised Janet because she'd never before experienced even a twinge of pain in her back. But if that was the problem, she wanted to get it fixed.

Unfortunately, to Janet's way of thinking, surgical fusion was not yet indicated. A more conservative course of therapy had to be tried. What about Back Power?

Test Results and Back Power Program

Janet's score on the tests was a *4* on the Sit-Up, indicating both significant stiffness in the back and, in her case, some discomfort in attempting to sit up. Straight Leg Raise scored *3*, which meant that Janet's stomach muscles were quite weak — most certainly the result of her two pregnancies and the fact that, between pregnancies, she had done nothing to improve muscle strength.

Sling muscles scored *1* on each side, a typical finding in most women; laterals scored *3* on the left and *1* on the right (for an average of 2). Janet's total was *10*.

With Janet's significant structural problem in her low back and loss of muscle strength, we gave her a modified Back Power program. Instead of doing Sit-Downs, which could aggravate her spondylolisthesis, she was to do a basic Curl exercise (to strengthen her stomach muscles) and, very gently, the Mad Cat (to improve flexibility in her back). The Sling Stretch was not indicated for Janet, but the Lateral Stretch and Lateral Leg Lift would improve her strength in this area.

Janet would still face a life of some back discomfort and pain, particularly on activity, but now she had a way of coping — of being the best she could possibly be. It gave Janet a measure of strength to know that she was in control to the best degree possible for her.

CASE HISTORY #5: TRAUMA TO LOW BACK

NAME: Angela

AGE: 49

At 49, Angela had fairly breezed through menopause. Unlike most of her friends, she hadn't experienced the irritability, hot flashes, and other complaints commonly associated with this condition. She felt very fortunate.

Going downstairs one day, Angela just missed the last step. Only a little stumble, but a sudden knife jab of pain in her lower lumbar spine literally caused her to collapse to the floor. Angela's husband helped her into a chair. The pain was unrelenting and became even worse with any attempt to move. Clearly, something serious had happened.

Angela was transported by ambulance to the emergency department at the local hospital. A brief examination followed by X-rays produced a diagnosis of a condition she'd read about but never associated with herself. In common with millions of women her age and older, Angela had osteoporosis, causing thinning and weakening of her vertebral bones. This had in turn caused a collapse of her L3 vertebral body when she slipped.

Though still in pain Angela felt reassured, knowing what was wrong, and that rest would help heal the fracture while painkillers as needed would make her comfortable. In eight to ten weeks, she'd be mobile again.

And mobile she was — *just*. Physically, Angela simply didn't feel the same. She had no stamina. Her back felt weak. But worse still, she lost confidence in herself. Angela knew that the osteoporosis had affected other vertebrae. She *feared* that each step she took could cause another problem.

Angela had heard about the controversy surrounding use of nutritional calcium supplements for osteoporosis. Whether or not these would help her, and regardless of the cost, she decided to try them. She even began to take more than the recommended daily dose "just in case." She seldom went out on her own any more.

Should Angela's life be transformed in this way — to one of fear and caution? Or could Back Power help?

Test Results and Back Power Program

A *4* on the Sit-Up test was the result of stiffness from Angela's fracture injury. On the Straight Leg Raise, Angela's score was *1*, but she scored a *4* on both the left sling and right lateral, indicating the contracture of her left side from muscle spasm caused by the trauma to that side of her back. Angela's total score on the tests was *12*.

Once the fracture was fully united, it left a significant structural weakness and change in the low back. Weak, unbalanced muscles holding up weakened bones only exacerbate the problem.

Angela was only too happy to take on the whole Back Power program to strengthen her back. In her case, too, a Curl was substituted for the Sit-Down exercise.

Angela persevered with her exercises and, in time, regained her self-confidence. Angela now has a part-time job at a local shopping center and makes a point of walking there and back. She does her Back Power exercises faithfully every day.

CASE HISTORY #6: DEGENERATIVE DISC DISEASE

NAME: Bill

AGE: 60

Bill emigrated from the United Kingdom more than 30 years ago, as a young man of 28. He had always been active, both at work as a police constable and in sports as a soccer player and swimmer. In the United Kingdom he played soccer on the local police team and had suffered one serious injury: a broken neck. Numerous small injuries included some damage to his knee cartilage, but he hadn't experienced any back pain or problems until he was about 40.

Then began a long history of nagging back pain that was diagnosed as degenerative disc disease. Bill's old sports injuries had healed in time, but his back pain only got worse. Numerous practitioners agreed there was nothing to be done except to live with the pain.

During the last six or seven years Bill's back became progressively worse. Bill has a house in the city as well as a summer cottage. His grass-cutting and handyman chores at both places keep him busy and active, but there were times when his back pain incapacitated him so that he couldn't function normally. Bill also had a fall at one point, which aggravated his problem.

As his bouts of back pain became more troublesome, Bill sought treatment. One specialist put him in a back brace, but Bill found he simply couldn't wear it. A surgeon who had Bill's back X-rayed stated that Bill "wasn't bad enough for surgery." Bill certainly didn't feel that way. He felt terrible.

Could Back Power help him?

Test Results and Back Power Program

Because of the stiffness associated with his age, Bill scored a *4* on the Sit-Up test. He'd already been doing stomach-strengthening exercises and a version of the Curl; as a result, he scored *2* on the Straight Leg Raise. Bill scored *3* on both left and right Sling tests and *4* on both of the Lateral tests. His total score was *13*. There was a lot of room for improvement.

Bill persevered at first with the Back Power exercise program, and some improvement was noted on the tests. He experienced great relief from back pain. Although he admits that at present he doesn't do his exercises daily, as he should, Bill does "rev himself up again" to do them at the first hint of any return of pain. "They've always worked for me," he says, "and that's better than any chemical prescription."

CASE HISTORY #7: METASTATIC DISEASE

NAME: Larry

AGE: 55

We had known Larry for several years. He was a safety professional at one of the companies we looked after, a man of about 55. We hadn't seen him for a while but remembered him as energetic and always cheerful. He'd not actually been a patient before and now, as he came in to our clinic, he looked sick. The usual smile was not there and there was no bounce in his gait. His face was pale and looked a bit thinner.

Larry sat down and explained that he'd had a nagging pain in his back for a couple of weeks and "it kind of worried" him. It was a pain that came on insidiously and he really couldn't understand why. He'd had no accident or injury, just this pain that came on one morning when he woke up. He said it wasn't affected by movement or rest. Larry had tried moving in various ways, but that made no difference. The one thing he did notice was that the pain got a lot worse at night — disturbing his sleep. He'd tried painkillers and found that aspirin with codeine helped a bit, but the pain seemed persistent and progressive.

Concerned at his mention of night pain, which can be a symptom of a serious disorder, we questioned Larry quite intensively about symptoms from other body organs. The only thing that he came up with was that he'd noticed a little slowing of his urine stream and a bit of burning too, particularly at night. Lately he'd had to get up to urinate during the night, something he never had to do in the past.

A very careful examination revealed nothing other than some localized tenderness in the low back. Because of Larry's urinary complaints, however, he was given a rectal examination — essential for proper assessment of a man his age. This confirmed our worst fears. The prostate gland, part of the urinary outflow from the kidneys, instead of being smooth and firm had a hard, angry nodule, which we knew had to be investigated further.

We referred Larry to a kidney specialist, who diagnosed cancer of the prostate, a relatively common type of cancer in men of Larry's age. Sadly, the cancerous nodule had grown beyond the prostate gland and metastasized, or spread, into the bones of his low back. That was what was causing his low back pain.

For Larry it was not just a question of having a problem diagnosed and then taking steps to rid himself of his low back pain. It was a question of struggling for life itself. With back pain, in most cases the cause is mechanical, muscular, or bony dysfunction. But every once in a while a Larry comes along to remind us that back pain is merely a symptom and that a high index of suspicion must always be there for more serious disorders of the body — particularly for first-time pain in a person over 50, and in particular where night pain is a prominent feature.

C.   Changing the Focus from Pain to Function

CASE HISTORY #8: "IT'S ALL IN THE MIND"
NAME: Susan
AGE: 27
Susan's situation was that of an individual with minimal organic pathology who had become severely disabled.

Her husband had phoned our clinic from the west to set up an appointment for her. He'd chronicled a tale of searching for help at a local university hospital, then at a respected institution in California, and later at a well-known clinic in the midwest. He'd heard positive reports about Back Power, and he wished to fly Susan in to see if our approach could help. They arrived, complete with Susan's vast medical history file and collection of X-rays.

Susan was now 27, with a two-year-old son at home. Her pain had begun during her pregnancy and gone away afterward, but then it returned a few months later, never to leave her. The pain had started in her low back but by now had spread to her whole back. She described jabbing here, numbness there, tingling and stinging somewhere else. It was quite a grab-bag of pains, but the bottom line was that Susan was *disabled by her pain.*

She had never returned to work since having the baby, even though the family needed the second income. She was virtually housebound. Her mother had moved in to help with the baby and with general chores. In short, Susan's functions as a mother, housewife, and companion were significantly reduced. Though she stated that she had resisted medication as she "didn't like taking drugs," Susan had become dependent on a number of proprietary drugs and the occasional prescription drug so that she could manage her pain. As Susan herself put it, her pain had become unbearable, *preventing* her from doing anything. *The pain prevented her!*

After listening to her story, we thumbed through the reams of information from three world-class institutions. She'd had every test in the book — not once or twice, but many times: X-rays, CATscan, magnetic resonance imagery (MRI), myelogram, bone scan. And though Susan had one or two abnormalities, each was prefaced with the word "slight." *Slight* change, *slight* elevation, *slight* abnormality, *slight* deviation from normal. . . .

She'd had every kind of treatment, too, one after the other: heat, rest, massage, brace, ultrasound, acupuncture, cortisone injections. None had lasting relief. Then came the final suggestion: that perhaps a psychological examination was in order.

Susan and her husband were unwilling to accept this recommendation. She'd been in good health before her back pain developed and had never shown signs of any psychological problems. They were convinced that there *must* be a mechanical reason for the problems in her low back.

We examined the patient, assessed the X-rays and various reports and, sure enough, there was no organic disability. The only significant finding was a number of fibrositic "trigger points" — small, tender nodules buried inside the muscle — which were exceedingly sensitive to the touch. These trigger points were distributed all over her body, with particular concentration around the spine.

How could a person become *so* disabled when there were so few organic findings?

Managing the Disability Process

Though our assessment of Susan agreed with all the others — that there were no structural abnormalities in the low back — a *functional* assessment showed significant loss of joint mobility at all levels of the spine as well as unbalanced, weak muscles. And significant dysfunction was indicated by the numerous trigger points throughout Susan's body. In addition, her pregnancy had resulted in a loosening of the pelvic ring, which meant that a pelvic stabilizing belt would be helpful.

When we explained the situation she was relieved, but at the same time she seemed somewhat disappointed that we hadn't found anything structurally wrong. Nevertheless, she listened intently as we outlined a course of action — something to *deal* with the problem. Susan was prepared to trust our evaluation and to give it her best in spite of pain, to exercise and balance her muscles, to strive for improved joint mobility. As well, the belt gave a sense of stability that she hadn't felt in several years. Susan seemed genuinely encouraged.

We'll never forget the way her husband's face lit up when we brought him back into the room and told him about our plans for treatment, which Susan had agreed to follow. He positively beamed as he told his wife to "wait right here while I go down and prepare the car."

We couldn't believe our ears. What he meant was that he was going down to rearrange the pillows he'd put in the back seat of the car so that Susan could ride back to their hotel in comfort. But we'd just finished telling him that there were no serious problems in her low back — that all she needed was some fresh air, exercise, and a little support. Here he was, still treating her like an invalid. In a desire to make her feel better, in his sympathy and concern for his wife, he was "enabling" and promoting Susan's disability behavior. He had missed the whole point. Susan needed to *push* herself. What dire consequences did he expect if she sat beside him, upright, in the front seat of the car in the normal way?

Susan did persist, though improvement took many months. As she gradually improved her muscle strength and balance, as her joints became more mobile, and as she began to regain confidence in herself, Susan's management of her problem started to *work*.

We saw her about a year later, and though she still had some discomfort she was progressing quite nicely.

"What *really* is the difference?" We asked her.

"Well, I thank *you*," she said, "because a year ago I was beginning to doubt myself — to wonder if I *did* have a mental problem of some sort. The difference now is that when I get back pain, instead of sitting down and putting my feet up, I go down to the Y, swim, and work it out. What's changed is not so much the pain as my reaction to it. Now I can help my*self*."

At last report, Susan's husband still cooks the family dinner. And Susan? She went back to work for a time, then went through a second pregnancy without difficulty. Her daily exercise program is now part of her life.

CASE HISTORY #9: A SELF-FULFILLING PROPHECY

NAME: Mario

AGE: 49

Like many before and many after him, Mario slowly pulled his way down the long corridor to our office. He came in, positioned himself by a chair, and slowly lowered his body into it. His face was expressionless as he waited for the question: "Mario, what seems to be the problem?"

After telling us that he had a pain in his back and showing the location with his hand, he finally said that he'd hurt his back 12 years previously. Mario was 49. He had been a manual laborer at the time of his injury.

Initially, Mario had put up with his back pain. When he finally consulted a specialist, he was admitted to a hospital and a myelogram was done.

"Yes, Mario, and what did they find?"

Sadly, with a quiet despair in his voice, he said: "They found that I was in such bad shape they couldn't operate. I'd end up a cripple."

Mario was discharged from the hospital, and his pain continued to distress him. He went back to work, but would be laid up periodically when the pain became unbearable. Still, on and off over those 12 years, Mario had persisted. His employer had cooperated by giving him lighter and lighter work, trying to help Mario carry on with life and to reduce the demands on his sick, "diseased" body. But finally the employer referred him to us because there were no more light jobs in the plant for Mario to do. His future employment picture looked bleak indeed.

Here was a man severely disabled in spite of his best attempts and his employer's. How did Mario get this way? Would anything work?

Managing the Disability Process

Mario was a first-generation immigrant to this country. His English was passable, but imperfect.

On investigation we found that the myelogram originally done on Mario had not indicated that his condition was too *bad* for surgery; rather, it had shown that there was no *indication* for surgery. This simple miscommunication had led him to behave for *12 years* as though the pain he felt was the *harm pain* that can produce a cripple, not the *hurt pain* that, in this case, was merely an indication of dysfunction: muscle imbalance and tightness, in the main. A miscommunication had become a self-fulfilling prophecy of disability.

Even so, Mario looked much younger that his stated years. On enquiry, I discovered that he'd come here originally as a professional soccer player. He'd been fit then, and strong, and his body still showed good form. His major problem was inflexibility — tightness in joints and muscles from years of athletic endeavor, years of hard work, and years of pain and spasm in his back.

As Mario began to deal with his dysfunction, using the daily exercise program we gave him, he began to make real progress and develop renewed self-confidence. Soon he was much more active, and when he returned to work it was in a role of greater productivity.

CASE HISTORY #10: A YOUNG MAN
KILLED WITH KINDNESS
NAME: Hal
AGE: 22

Hal was a young, strong, physical specimen, but at 22 years of age he'd come seeking help. He was about to lose his job — a well-paid job with a future, one he wanted to keep.

Several years before, Hal had started to develop the typical pattern of ankylosing spondylitis: stiffness in the morning, which went away as the day progressed. Gradually, though, the symptoms became unbearable and Hal sought relief — first through over-the-counter medications and heat, then from a health professional.

It didn't take long for his doctor to make a diagnosis. Stiffness and tenderness of the back, combined with X-rays showing the minor changes of *sclorosis* (darkening around the sacroiliac joints) and elevated blood tests, indicated arthritis.

Hal's response to medication was good but by no means perfect, and he was still disabled by a significant amount of pain. His doctor had requested that Hal's employer give him a lighter-duty job, but the employer had no other work (apart from his own) that would be suitable for Hal. He suggested that Hal find other employment if he could not carry on.

Hal was angry at his employer's response because he'd already given him a number of good years and had, in fact, once injured his back on one job, further aggravating his problem. Hal felt that he was owed something and that he was being treated in a shabby way.

Managing the Disability Process

Quite clearly, Hal had received good medical assessment and care. He'd had the proper diagnosis and had been encouraged to be active and maintain joint mobility with the right kind of exercises. Hal had also been prescribed anti-inflammatory medication, and physiotherapy had been arranged for him.

But, two things upset Hal. First, his doctor, though well-meaning, had arranged for assessment by the local arthritic society for "supportive care." Here was Hal, a vital 22-year-old with some arthritis in his spine, being visited by a representative from the arthritic society as if he were an invalid. What message did this convey to Hal? What future was in store for him? How bad were things going to get?

Second, the doctor had made this recommendation: "He can no longer maintain his present occupation, which requires a lot of physical activity. Even though physical activity is desirable, the degree of labor that he performs is *probably* too severe for him to sustain in his present condition."

Well-meaning advice, well-meaning arrangements for supportive care, but in both cases killing a patient with kindness. In fact, physical activity was *very* desirable — the more the better, to create greater mobility in the low back. The doctor had made *his* suggestion not on the basis of what was necessary, but on the basis of his own *assumption* that the patient was unwilling to cope with some hurt pain, even for benefit, and that this patient had to be babied.

By so doing, Hal's doctor had made a decision that only the patient himself could make. This was a personal choice, *not* a medically indicated choice.

CASE HISTORY #11: "THERE MUST BE SOMETHING WRONG!"

NAME: Gus

AGE: 36

Gus was a 36-year-old laborer who enjoyed his work and had been with his company for almost 20 years.

His work was recognized as good, he was conscientious, and he got on well with people. Many times he had been offered promotion to supervisory work but he'd resisted because he *liked* manual labor — liked to be outside in the fresh air and sunshine, enjoyed the feel of the earth between his shovel and his foot. For Gus, a promotion to supervisor, although paying better money, would be a poorer quality of life. Unfortunately, something had come to darken the picture.

Over the past few years, Gus had developed recurrent bouts of back pain, which were becoming more and more persistent. He'd sought various forms of treatment — from physiotherapists, chiropractors, and physicians. The last physician had told Gus that his back was degenerating, that the discs were wearing out, and that if he continued in his present occupation, he'd be "burnt out" in a very few years. That's when he came to see us.

Could anything be done to slow the process and maintain the quality of life he wished?

Managing the Disability Process

Although Gus had been advised that he'd become a low-back cripple if he continued his laboring job, results of his examination from each doctor had been normal. There was no tenderness, and Gus had a full range of movement in his back. The only positive finding had been diagnosis of slight arthritis (degenerative discs) on the X-rays, although two years later another radiologist read Gus's X-rays as showing normal. The first radiologist, it would seem, had overread the X-rays to find a "cause."

The diagnosis from Gus's last specialist was unequivocal, however:

> **I think it is clear that this gentleman is telling of a job-related polyarthralgia and further, his whole problem is job-related and it is compensatable if he ever wants to approach the insuring agency. In the meantime, he is earning a very good income if he simply pushes himself harder and harder. I've offered him a list of analgesics that I've asked him to take pill for pill with a Tagamet.**

> This is a sad situation. He has had many years with this company and
> is very experienced but there seems to be no program for advancement.
> In short, ten years from now, he may still be doing the same job and
> complaining even more. A sad situation.

Was it any wonder that Gus was so upset? First, he was told he had
a polyarthralgia. That just means he had many pains in the joints. It is
not a medical diagnosis, but it frightened the life out of Gus. He
thought he had a terminal disease.

The examination had shown nothing wrong, but rather than stating
this fact it was thought better to give an explanation for the *pain* — a
classic example of labeling the pain symptom as though it were a disease.

Next, Gus was offered treatment for the *pain* in the form of analgesics,
which were taken "pill for pill" with Tagamet, an anti-ulcer medication.
Instead of having one type of medication, Gus had been given one for the
pain, another to counteract the side effects of the first.

Rather than receiving concrete advice in terms of how he could
function better to maintain his situation, Gus got a litany of sympathy,
reproach for his employer, and the suggestion to go on compensation
— to become even *more* disabled.

We provided Gus with an exercise program, which he includes in
his daily routine. This routine has made a world of difference, and Gus
still resists that promotion in favor of the work he so enjoys.

CASE HISTORY #12: THE SHOW MUST GO ON
NAME: Rita
AGE: 30

Rita, a 30-year-old professional writer, always enjoyed sports. She
kept in shape at a fitness club and jogged and swam regularly. She
was, in short, the picture of good health.

One day, Rita had just completed a session at her typewriter, and as
she stood up she felt a sudden, sharp pain down her leg, almost throw-
ing her off balance. Realizing that this was no ordinary pain — especially when it began to get worse — Rita made her way to the emergency department at the local hospital. She was limping slightly, bent
forward, and tilted to one side in her pain. After examination and X-
rays (which were normal), findings showed weakness in the right
ankle and right leg along with diminished reflex and limitation in the
Straight Leg Raise. All signs pointed to an acute herniated disc.

Rita was told to go home, rest for a week, and take analgesics — to put her feet up and take it easy. This was not going to be easy: not only had Rita never been inactive for that long in her life, she was self-employed and had no sickness benefits or other source of income. The degree of pain, however, convinced her that she must follow the advice she'd been given. She really didn't have much choice.

Follow-up examination one week later showed the presence of findings of herniated disc, but the pain was beginning to settle down and Rita's doctor gave the go-ahead for a gradual increase in activity. Manuscript deadlines and the sheer necessity of "keeping the wolf from the door" meant that Rita was willing to pay the pain price and continue with her life as best she could. As a writer, her motto was "the show must go on."

I saw Rita several weeks later on referral from her physician. Could her pain situation be improved?

Managing the Disability Process

After our consultation, Rita was given some gentle stretching exercises that began to loosen up the tight muscles and improve the biomechanics of her back. She was to do this stretching several times a day.

Gradually, the findings for the herniated disc began to recede. As the disc slowly repaired itself, more exercises were added until Rita's back function was restored to being as good as it could possibly be.

Here was the case of an individual who had a significant, serious disorder, managed it well, understood the ramifications of her condition — the difference between *hurt* and *harm* pain — and was prepared to take an active role to maintain function while she was getting better, then *restore* function when appropriate.

Throughout the whole course of her problem, this individual with a serious back disorder was disabled for only one week and seriously hampered for only a few weeks.

11

Answering Your Questions

About Back Problems

I've been told my back problem was caused by lumbar strain/ degenerative disc disease/osteoporosis/facet syndrome/scoliosis. What will Back Power do for me?

For any pain disorder, prudence dictates guidance and advice from your health practitioner, and in your situation Back Power tests and exercises can be customized for your individual needs. Except for serious diseases, Back Power, when the acute problem is under control, will usually eliminate or at least minimize your problem.

- *Lumbar strain* is a nonspecific term referring to minimal organic clinical findings, no signs of nerve root irritation, and no internal disease. X-rays are normal. The Back Power program is usually a major help.

- *Degenerative disc disease* has similar findings but usually occurs in an older age group. (We consider the term to be a misnomer; disc degeneration is a normal part of the aging process.) X-rays show some aging and arthritic changes, although most people with this condition have developed the normal aging that appears after age 40. The Back Power tests and exercises provide maximum muscular support, minimizing weak bony support.

- *Osteoporosis* is a weakened condition of the bony support of the spine caused by loss of calcium, the material that strengthens bone. This condition is discovered by X-ray. It often causes partial collapse of one or more vertebral bodies. Although osteoporosis is more common in women (caused by hormonal changes at menopause), it is sometimes found in older men as well. Many practitioners now recommend regular *gentle* movement and exercise, which seem to improve calcium deposit in the bone. Back Power can be customized to your needs by your health professional, ensuring safety and effectiveness.

- *Facet syndrome* is a condition of discomfort in the back caused by weight-bearing on the facet joints instead of on the vertebral body. Discomfort is increased by bending your back in extension (backward). Many facet syndromes are caused by imbalance of supporting muscles (tight sling muscles, weak abdominals) and can be improved by Back Power.
- *Scoliosis* is a curve in the spine laterally. Although scoliosis can be caused by bony changes, much of the effect of the condition can be corrected or improved by improving the balance of the supporting trunk muscles, especially the sling and lateral muscles.

I've had surgery. What precautions should I take when trying the Back Power tests and exercises?

After recovery from back surgery, rehabilitation of weak supporting trunk muscles is essential. Your surgeon knows your personal needs and problems and should provide personal guidance in customizing the program and introducing each exercise in the proper sequence and at the proper speed.

Would Back Power help my sciatica problem?

Sciatica is a description of pain that localizes in one or both legs and may radiate down to the foot and toes. Sciatica may be accompanied by weakness of muscles and diminishment or loss of reflexes. It is usually caused by pressure on a nerve root that supplies one or both legs. This pressure in turn is most commonly caused by a herniated disc, spinal stenosis, or a narrowing of the intervertebral foramen.

Following proper diagnosis and conservative care, Back Power can be a major help in the rehabilitation process. Because this is a disease situation, you should, however, have personal advice from your health professional. He or she will suggest the appropriate Back Power exercises, tell you how often you should do them, and grade them according to your needs.

About the Back Power Tests and Exercises

Why is it that exercise makes my back feel worse?

This situation often occurs because the back is the foundation of all movement. A weak foundation is aggravated by manual work, sports, and other exercise that involves the arms and legs, but the Back Power approach is different.

The tests identify specific weaknesses and imbalance in the trunk and spinal muscles. Once these are known, an exercise program can be customized to balance your trunk muscles. This approach gives you a much better chance to reach your full potential in exercise and to live life the way you want. The key point about Back Power is that it loosens tight muscles and tightens long muscles. It isn't just "any old exercise" for all backs but a specific individual program based on your test score. That is why Back Power offers a high success rate and diminishes back pain.

We should note that some discomfort in the initial stages is quite normal. This situation results from what we call the "progressive overload" principle, which means that when you begin to exercise a muscle that's out of shape, some discomfort or overload can be expected.

Why do you emphasize a relaxed breathing technique?

For maximum benefit from the Back Power program, you must develop the skill of relaxed breathing. Many people neglect this skill because they judge it too easy, a waste of time, or something they've done all their lives and needn't practice.

A deep, slow breath in, followed by a relaxed exhalation, causes a relaxation message to go from your brain to your muscles. This breathing pattern sets up a relaxation response in the muscles, permitting them to elongate to their naturally healthy length without pain or discomfort. Most patients agree that, second to the Back Power tests, the most important thing about the program is the breathing. Relaxed breathing is what makes the exercise program so effective.

The Back Power exercises seem so simple. How can they work?

The Back Power program *is* simple. It works because the Back Power tests identify your area (or areas) of weakness and then emphasize exactly the kind of exercise you need: stretch-relaxation to lengthen weak, tight muscles; power-stretch exercises to shorten long, flabby muscles that are also weak. Five minutes devoted daily in a consistent manner is all most people need to be the best they can possibly be.

Back Power — when should I do it? how often? how many repetitions?

We recommend the best time to do Back Power exercises is first thing in the morning, when you roll out of bed. First, the exercises help to wake you up and make you more alert; second, this is the time when you may be at your worst — when you're stiff. You'll also find that the Back Power/Muscle Maintenance program is helpful as a warm-up before sports or other activities, such as gardening.

We recommend that the Back Power exercises be done once a day, though some people like to do them before going to bed as well. We suggest that each stretch-relaxation exercise be done three times, each power-strength exercise five to ten times. It's easy — and what seems to work best for most people. All you need is five minutes daily for the regular Back Power exercises, and ten minutes for the Muscle Maintenance program.

Is Muscle Maintenance all the exercise I need?

True fitness is a combination of the four S's:

- slimness,
- stamina,
- strength,
- suppleness.

Slimness means weight control. *Stamina* means endurance and cardiovascular fitness — the ability of the heart to pump sufficient oxygen to the muscles. Muscle Maintenance looks after *strength* and *suppleness* for the major muscle groups in your trunk, spine, arms, and legs.

Full fitness also requires an endurance program such as swimming, walking, or jogging. Taken together, Muscle Maintenance and an aerobic exercise will see you well on the way to a balanced fitness program.

I was told never to do a sit-up. What do you recommend?

It's important to differentiate between the two types of sit-up. One is done by locking the feet under a bed or sofa — having them anchored in some way. This sit-up is primarily an exercise for the sling muscles, and it can aggravate a weak back or put it at risk.

Back Power does use a sit-up test *once*, to determine the level of flexibility in the low back. Our sit-up method is of the second type, where the feet are *not* anchored. We then use a sit-down exercise that helps to strengthen and tighten loose stomach muscles. Curling back slowly without anchoring the feet has, in our experience, proven an effective exercise with very low risk.

Some conditions such as spondylolisthesis and pelvic ring disorders *can* be aggravated by the sit-down exercises. In these cases, we recommend the Curl exercise exclusively.

If your health professional has recommended that you never do a sit-up, replace it with the Curl, which is almost as effective.

I know I shouldn't bounce when I stretch, so why have I been told that the stretch-and-hold technique is best?

Bouncing, of course, stimulates the muscle spindles to "fire," resulting in tightening of the muscles. The stretch-and-hold technique is practiced by many athletes and involves stretching the muscle to its maximum length and holding for 20 to 30 seconds. This is indeed an excellent way to stretch a muscle. Back Power uses the stretch-and-hold technique along with the relaxed breathing technique, which enhances the stretch and permits it to occur in a shorter time period.

I've been told never to do the Double Leg Raise exercise. Do you agree?

This is excellent advice. The Double Leg Raise is a very risky exercise, even for people with a good back. For those with a weak back it can be a serious source of problems.

We use the Double Leg Raise as a test, *not* an exercise, to be done once and stopped as soon as the back arches off the floor. The Double Leg Raise provides a good indication of stomach muscle strength — but it's a very poor exercise.

I get enough exercise at work. Why do I need Back Power?

Back Power is essential to restore a back to its optimal health and strength. The back and trunk musculature is different from the muscles in the arms and legs. Back muscles are like four strands in a rope: they work together and are called *synergistic* (*syn* = together, *ergon* = work). When injury causes contraction of one or more muscles in the trunk, work will not restore length and balance; instead, it will cause overuse and aggravation of the normal, healthy muscles. The only way to restore synergistic muscles to normal is to isolate each muscle group in its place of action and then give the appropriate exercise: strengthening or stretching.

I've been told that all exercise should incorporate the pelvic tilt. The Mad Cat exercise has an extension phase that conflicts with this caution. Why?

The Mad Cat stretch exercise has been used for centuries as part of yoga technique. Although extension was a concern several years ago, physiotherapists during the past few years have championed the extension technique developed by Robin Mackenzie. They've used this technique successfully in treating acute pain. The purpose of the Back Power program is to restore a normal range of movement to the spine, which includes both flexion and extension. The Mad Cat stretching exercise is an essential and necessary part of the program.

I've tried the Sling Stretch and felt discomfort in the base of my spine over the sacroiliac joints. What should I do?

This is an important exercise, particularly for young people and especially for athletic men and women. As people age, however there is more likelihood of looseness in the pelvic ring. The Sling Stretch, if pursued too aggressively, not only creates looseness of the sling muscles but can aggravate and cause looseness in the pelvic ring in general and the sacroiliac joints in particular.

If you feel discomfort in this area, you should stop the Sling Stretch for a week or two. Then try it again, experiment with wearing the Back Power belt as you do it, and make sure you pursue this exercise at a less intense level.

The Lateral Lift looks very difficult. Should I be afraid to try it?

The Lateral Lift is not an exercise. It's a test of lateral muscle strength. Many people think that it's difficult, then find it quite easy — as long as it's done properly. Lateral muscles are the most neglected of the four types of trunk muscles, and for this reason we urge you to try this test. The Lateral Lift often demonstrates the greatest deficiency, and it can be an indicator of how you can achieve the most improvement.

I know I have a weak back, but I think I'll leave well enough alone because I've had so much trouble. Shouldn't I be afraid?

The Back Power program is to help people strengthen a weak back — to be the best they can possibly be — but you are a free agent, of course, and must make a personal choice and commitment. Some people have had so much trouble with their back that they rightly recognize a degree of risk and are often afraid to start the program. Life is, however, filled with risk/reward equations. A weak spine held up by weak muscles is a sure recipe for trouble. Back Power is about minimizing your trouble by supporting the weak spine with strong back muscles.

Are you prepared to take a risk to experience the reward of being the best you can possibly be? In order to improve your chances, get advice from your health professional, then start the program — gradually.

Are the Back Power exercises all right for children to do?

Although few children complain of back pain and our major experience is with adults, it's surprising how soon trunk muscles can tighten up and become weak — even in children. We're told that the maximum degree of fitness in the young is reached somewhere between the ages of 10 and 13. We've found the Back Power tests a unique way to get children's attention and improve their interest in fitness generally — stressing the importance of keeping their muscles strong and balanced. The tests customize the program for each individual.

I've been told not to jog or participate in sports. What level of exercise can I do?

Back problems result from a mismatch between the task attempted and the capability of the individual. Unfortunately, the normal approach to minimizing back problems is to minimize activity — whether work or play — thereby diminishing enjoyment of life. Back Power was designed to increase the capability of the individual so that he or she can enjoy a fuller life.

Don'ts reduce your chance of risk in the environment, but we like to emphasize *do's* that improve your individual capability.

No one can say with certainty what level of activity is for you. The only way to know is to is to be the best you can possibly be — to find out for yourself.

What about yoga?

Muscles tighten up and become short through injury, stress, aging and, paradoxically, excessive manual labor or exercise. In Eastern cultures, the tradition of stretching — yoga, tai-chi, the Japanese martial arts — has become fully ingrained as a necessary life skill. This is not the case in Western societies, however, causing many people to develop tight muscles — particularly after age 30.

Stretch-relaxation exercise is very similar to yoga but has been simplified, making it much easier for North Americans to be introduced to the concept of stretching, to feel its benefits and, for many, to get coaching in a full yoga program at a later date.

Are back extension exercises good for people with back problems?

The basic rule that dominates Back Power is balance: balance of joint movement (neither too little nor too much); balance of muscles for optimal health and strength (not too short and not too long). The aim of Back Power is to identify needs in terms of lack of joint movement and lack of muscle balance, and so provide a program to support those needs.

If you lack extension range of movement, extension exercises are usually of significant benefit. On the other hand, if you lack flexion movement, then flexion movements and exercises are required. The basic rule is to define what *you* need, not to subscribe dogmatically to one type of exercise or another.

About the Back Power Belt

If I use the Back Power belt, will my muscles weaken?

The Back Power belt is an intertrochanteric belt, which means that it stabilizes bones and ligaments and has very little effect on muscles. The belt is recommended only for a two- to three-week period and only in conjunction with rehabilitation exercises to restore muscle balance. The Back Power belt is a temporary adjunct to management, much as a cast or splint helps in the healing of a fracture. It is a means to an end, not an end in itself.

I have a specific *problem — degeneration of the L5/S1 disc — and a positive Chair test. What does this mean?*

As mentioned in chapter 4, having a specific problem such as degeneration of a disc is often not the total problem. A positive Chair test can indicate dysfunction in the pelvic ring, which can cause or be caused by other problems, such as your disc problem. For this reason, you should read chapter 6 on the pelvic ring disorders and get advice on how to act accordingly.

I don't like anything artificial. The Chair test is positive, the belt helps, but I'd prefer living with the problem. What do you think?

The Back Power belt, as mentioned, is like a cast or a splint — it's a device to help improve low back function and provide a strong pelvic foundation. As with the whole Back Power program, a decision must be based on weighing the benefits of wearing the belt against the "risks." Experience has shown that the belt is highly effective in stabilizing the pelvic ring. Without accomplishing this stability, people tend to have chronic recurring problems for the rest of their lives. Again, as with the whole program, it's personal choice and commitment that count. We respect your right to make your own choice.

When I move or do certain exercises, there is a click in my back. What causes this? Will the Back Power belt help?

There are many reasons given for the audible click or clunk in the low back. In our experience, a click usually indicates instability somewhere in the pelvic ring. You should read chapter 6 on the pelvic ring disorders and follow its lead.

We've found that the belt and stabilizing exercises often do not correct this problem. When an audible click is present, we advise people to use the Curl instead of the sit-down exercise and caution against aggressive stretching of the sling muscles. The click tends to indicate a negative prognosis and the possibility of recurrence in the future. With the Back Power program, however, you'll be able to minimize recurrences as much as is possible.

About Chiropractors

What is adjustment?

The goal of smooth back function is normal movement of joints at individual vertebral levels along with balance and strength in the supporting musculature. When a health professional assesses the spine for function, both manually and through motion X-rays, he or she can define a locking or lack of movement at certain levels of the spine. Lack of movement at one level tends to put strain and stress on other levels of the spine, causing excessive movement at these other levels.

An adjustment, or manipulation, is a manual maneuver used by chiropractors to move the blocked segment and create normal movement. Chiropractors prefer the term "adjustment" because it signifies something more skilled, more precise, and less forceful than manipulation. It is interesting to note that forms of manipulation are also used by osteopaths and a small group of physicians practicing orthopedic medicine, and that a variation called mobilization, which causes slightly less movement, is used by a small group of specially trained physiotherapists.

Although adjustment or manipulation is not limited to the chiropractic profession, chiropractors have the most extended and specialized training in this area of health care.

How well are chiropractors trained?

Chiropractors, like physicians, are required to complete a premedical course — usually they have a Bachelor of Science — at an accredited university. The chiropractic course itself is a four-year course covering in-depth anatomy, pathology, physics — all the basic sciences covered by a physician, with the exception of pharmacology.

Chiropractic education is controlled by international accreditation standards and has been found by a number of independent government inquiries to be the equivalent of undergraduate medical education. In some specialized areas, such as radiology, there is more concentrated and detailed training than at medical college.

Chiropractors are specifically trained to identify diseases that are beyond their scope of practice, such as internal diseases causing low back pain, and refer patients to a physician. A number of independent inquiries affirm the ability to diagnose and the general high standards and safety of chiropractic medicine.

Why do chiropractors take so many X-rays?

As with any tests, the use of X-rays must be balanced against the value or benefit they give for diagnosis and the risks — in this case, the risk of radiation. A chiropractor takes the normal set of X-rays to determine structural abnormalities in the low back but often adds motion X-rays. These help to define locked segments in the spine which are amenable to adjustment or other manual therapy.

About Medication

I don't like taking painkillers, but sometimes I really need them. What should I do?

Sometimes the pain becomes so intense that painkillers are required. It's most important first to have a proper diagnosis to determine that the increased pain is not related to a serious disorder, and that your activity level is appropriate for your particular problem. In general, painkillers are not recommended for daytime activities, though some type of anti-pain prescription may be given if necessary so that people can get as normal a night's sleep as possible. Abnormal sleep patterns night after night can otherwise accelerate depression and discourage the patient.

The important thing to note about painkillers is that they must not be taken as an end in themselves. They do not treat the basic condition causing the pain but are rather another means to an end: they make the patient more comfortable while he or she is getting better and undertaking physical therapy.

What do anti-inflammatory pills do?

These pills — which include aspirin, other nonprescription medications, and prescription medications — possess an anti-inflammatory action that can be highly effective, particularly in ankylosing spondylitis and other problems involving inflammatory arthritis. In these conditions, they are part of the treatment and should not be avoided if prescribed but taken on a regular basis. In reducing inflammation, they also reduce pain and permit the patient to become more active, if that is desirable.

What is the purpose of heat, cold, massage, acupuncture, ultrasound, and other such treatments?

Many people regard these treatments (and others) as ends in themselves. In the Back Power program, we believe that they, like painkillers, are adjuncts to treatment. While Back Power is restoring movement to joints and balance to muscles, such treatments can make the patient more comfortable, reducing pain levels.

There is much controversy over the use of *heat* and *massage* as a therapy. In general, we use *cold* where there has been an acute injury or trauma to the back and where we suspect stretching of ligaments, straining of muscles, and possible internal bleeding. Cold helps to constrict the blood vessels, limiting the amount of internal bleeding as well as being a counterirritant to help reduce pain.

In general, cold is used in the initial phase of the injury. After 48 hours or with acute muscle spasm or strain, we use heat to improve the blood supply and reduce spasm and pain in surrounding muscles and tissues.

Massage in all its forms is helpful, too, in improving blood supply, particularly to short, spasmed muscles — so permitting better range of movement for the underlying joints.

Acupuncture, acupressure, and other forms of this treatment usually are applied to areas where fibrositis or trigger-points exist. Acupuncture is a good form of pain relief, but in most cases its effect is temporary. Time and comfort gained by this form of pain relief, especially in chronic conditions, permit the patient to restore joint movement and balance muscles. Acupuncture's value is as a means to an end, not as an end in itself.

Ultrasound and other more sophisticated physical therapy treatments help to reduce deep-seated inflammation in muscles, ligaments, and joints and can be an important adjunct to overall treatment aims.

About External Factors

How much should a person lift?

It has proven impossible to develop a standard for a maximum acceptable lift. Each person has different capabilities, and as we've seen, back injury results from a mismatch between these capabilities and the demands of the task. The individual capabilities in turn depend on strength of the bones, the discs, and the muscles of the back. The Back Power program helps maximize individual strengths as much as is possible.

We do note that any discussion of weight-bearing must include not only the *weight of the object* being moved but also the *distance* moved, the height and *position* from which the object is moved, the distance away from the body when carried, the *repetition* factor, and many other factors. So it is that no set answer can be given except that in general, the greater the load, the greater the risk to the majority of people.

What do you think about waterbeds?

Most people who use a waterbed find that it helps to reduce stiffness and discomfort upon waking in the morning. The whole approach to the Back Power program, however, is not to baby one's back with a special bed, but to restore one's back capability to health and strength as much as possible. That would be the time to think about buying a waterbed.

Waterbeds work by permitting passive, gentle movements during the night rather than one static position. The same effect can be accomplished with a firm mattress, which helps to promote movement and different positions throughout the night, thus reducing stiffness and immobility the next morning. The worst kind of mattress is one that sags — where a person tends to stay in one position over long periods, with resulting stiffness and loss of motion on waking.

What kind of shoes should I wear to help my back?

As with the waterbed, we advise that first you strengthen your back to its maximum capability — be the best you can be. We do not recommend buying special shoes or other adjuncts to "take the pressure off" a weak back. In general, however, high-heeled shoes tend to alter the posture and aggravate lordosis in the low back, as well as facet syndrome, and in many cases these two disorders can be improved by backward-tilting Earth shoes. But again: why baby a weak back? Why not restore your back to normal — and have a better chance of wearing the kinds of shoes you prefer?

Can clothing aggravate a bad back?

In some cases, where a great deal of movement is involved in a task, tight-fitting pants may prevent proper biomechanics and lifting techniques, so producing excessive strains and possible injury in the low back.

What if my job itself or a poor workplace design is the cause of my problem?

Back problems are the result of that mismatch between the individual's capabilities and the demands of the task or environment. Back Power addresses the individual. But a proper approach to back problems must, of course, involve identifying risks in tasks and the environment, and reducing these risks through proper workplace design. The study of the relationship between people and their workplace is called *ergonomics*. Its application is becoming increasingly widespread, promising better design in everyday environments to improve human performance and reduce unnecessary stress and strain on the spinal column and on the body in general.

Challenging the Traditional

Challenging Your Perspective

As we've shown throughout our book, building Back Power has meant challenging the accepted views of looking at back problems. Our approach challenges the traditional views in a number of important ways. *By reversing the notion that the back is fragile, weak, vulnerable to the slightest injury; that it is a structure that must be pampered by way of a multitude of don'ts (don't lift, don't jog, don't do anything active).* Back Power defines the back as strong, resilient, and indeed *powerful* — an intricate engineering miracle with many parts that, complex as they are, have been designed to work beautifully together. The back that has *become* weakened as the result of dysfunction, disease, or injury is not a structure to pamper and ignore. Rather, reconditioning and strengthening are the keys.

Hence, our Back Power motto: "To give you the information — the opportunity — to be the best you can be."

By looking at back pain, the symptom, and defining it on three levels:

1) *harm* pain — the structural disease level — corrected by treatment intervention;
2) *hurt* pain — the dysfunctional level — corrected by a combination of treatment and the patient's personal effort;
3) pain as the *cause of disability* — the behavioral level — which can only be managed through an individual's personal choice, with action based on sound information.

By developing a clear model — the Back Power functional model — based on balance: balance of joints in the spine and balance of sup-

porting musculature. Such a model forms the basis of a reconditioning and rehabilitation program that encourages a consistent and rational approach and relegates pain treatment to a secondary role.

By placing a primary emphasis (1) on prevention and (2) on a management plan that complements diagnosis and treatment.

By teaching management of the disability process and by combining treatment with personal, active involvement spurred by personal choice.

By correctly defining back pain. Most people suffering from back-ache are diagnosed as having a lumbar strain, a facet syndrome, or some other imprecise ailment. Is this approach scientific? Is it *really* a diagnosis? Or is it a name for pain, which then permits the focus to be on treatment of that pain — treatment of a *symptom.*

Most back pain is caused by mechanical dysfunction, and it follows that the goal in treatment and management of the problem must be to restore normal function by promoting normal joint movement and balanced supporting musculature. Chemical (drug) treatment to modify pain must assume a secondary role.

Challenging the Cost of Back Injuries

Although a cost estimate relative to back injuries is hard to arrive at, these most recent statistics provide a sense of the magnitude of such costs.

- In the United States, total annual direct Workers' Compensation Board (WCB) payments amount to *$10 billion.*
- In the United Kingdom, these annual payments are £1,000 million.
- In Canada, the annual total is $1 billion.
- For time lost because of back injury, the annual worker average in Canada is 53 days.
- In North America, the average *initial* cost per back injury has been calculated at $5,480.
- For a *settled* claim, the North American average is $30,000-$100,000 (figure includes pension payments).
- Indirect costs resulting from lost productivity, including the expense of worker replacement and training, are *in addition* many times the actual WCB costs.
- The incidence of back pain per 100,000 workers has risen from 210 in 1960 to 717 in 1980.

These commonly cited costs refer only to *first* injuries, but of course back problems recur. As for the indirect WCB cost factor, in Canada these costs approach $4 billion annually; in the United States, $40-$50 billion.

Emphasis on dollars and cents often obscures a hidden cost: the personal price of back injury. As stated in *The Hidden Epidemic: Back Injuries*, a pamphlet produced by one of the largest unions in North America:

> Clearly, the economic cost of this epidemic is unacceptable, the cost in human suffering is incalculable and intolerable. The pain suffered, the loss of mobility, the loss of shared family pleasures, the loss of self-esteem for those put out of work. These are the uncounted costs paid by the injured workers and their families.

Back problems strike working people at the rate of 1.5-2.0 per 100 workers per year. But these statistics relate only to *working people on compensation*. They do not reflect medical, drug, hospital, and lost-time costs for non-work-related injury.

Statistical trends indicate that back problems are increasing, lasting longer, costing more, being treated with more drugs, and disabling more people than ever before. During the past decade in Canada, the number of treatments for physical therapy has increased 400 percent, with only marginal population growth. Quite a paradox at a time when we are better fed, clothed, housed than ever before and our work has become more automated, imposing fewer physical demands.

Yet with all the suffering, all the activity, and all the costs, the total funds allocated to prevention — real *health* care expenditures — are less than 2 percent of total *disease* care expenditures. Little prevention funding is directed toward the problem back; rather, it is channeled to the more life-threatening cancer, heart disease and, now, AIDS.

A Balanced Approach

Outlook

Most people, when questioned, blame their back problem on something *external* (my shoes, my chair, my bed, my job) or on their having done something wrong (I lifted or twisted the wrong way, I slipped and fell). As pointed out in our book, there is a significant need to identify risks in the task, in the work place, and in the environment, to minimize these risks in any way possible, and to eliminate risks whenever that is possible.

But balance is necessary. Back Power can help you to balance the risk equation by identifying *risk in yourself*. The Back Power tests show whether your back is weak and unbalanced and so prone to injury. The Back Power exercises can help you to strengthen — to balance — your back to lessen the risk of an injury and avoid the all-too-common cycle of:

weak back → injury → weaker back→ more susceptible to another injury.

Self-Reliance and Treatment

Give a man a fish and he'll be hungry tomorrow.
Teach a man to fish and he'll never be hungry.

— Chinese proverb

With back pain, the major emphasis in the past has been on treating the pain experience with mood-altering chemicals. This approach follows the "if it hurts, don't do it" school of thought. A recent study in the *New England Journal of Medicine* gave cause for reflection about this topic. Its conclusion? That after a back injury, two days' bed rest followed by appropriate activity produced better results in most people than seven days' bed rest. Less is more.

Prevention involves giving people the tools to cope — knowledge, skills, coaching — but expecting them to take active steps to manage their own back problem. As one practitioner wrote to us, "All doctors agree with your basic approach of getting the back patient involved with care of his or her own back. The question is how to do it."

Although most health practitioners agree that fitness and movement are necessary for back health, the most *frequent* response we hear from them is, "Yes, but people won't do it. When the pain goes away, they forget about their backs. They won't keep up with an exercise program." This argument is not valid. What about the decision an individual must make to keep fit? To stop smoking? To limit or eliminate alcohol consumption? To ensure proper nutrition for self and family? Some do. Some don't. All deserve the opportunity to make their personal decision.

A failure to emphasize prevention and personal responsibility in the management of back problems can only result in further escalation of health care costs for the minority — unnecessary, wasteful costs — and thereby rationing of care for the majority.

High Tech, Low Tech

The further we proceed into the age of high technology, the more aware we become of the limitations of high-tech solutions.

In medicine, the recent discovery that ASA (aspirin, or acetylsalicylic acid) taken every other day helps reduce the risk of heart attack is very much on the *low-tech* side. ASA, the first synthetic drug, was developed more than a hundred years ago. Balance its cost (pennies) against that of a heart transplant (about $150,000) — a high-tech solution — and we have *im*balance.

High-tech surgical and drug treatment are costly and can make dramatic impact. Low-tech movement and exercise done daily can have a major impact as well — just as low-tech daily brushing of teeth complements high-tech dental equipment and procedures.

Another feature of today's high-tech testing capacity is that our ability to define problems by these means has outstripped our ability to interpret abnormalities.

The CATscan, for instance, is a sophisticated tool that can now identify "bulging discs" in the low back — something that could never be done as easily before. The problem is that 25 percent of "normal" people without any back pain show these "bulging discs." Is this a normal aging process that should be left alone? Or is it pathology that needs cutting out? The problem is further complicated because CATscans are ordered only for chronic back pain sufferers; a large enough number of nonpain "normals" is lacking for comparison. This situation could cause overinterpretation of results and unnecessary surgery.

In building Back Power, we've tried to combine the best of both worlds, being conscious of the costs and the limitations of high tech and appreciative of an increasing public demand for a return to the art of healing: the compassionate, hands-on, caring approach.

Financial Compensation

Organic pathology in the spine can now be defined with a high degree of accuracy. Functional impairment can be determined with reasonable certainty. But disability — low back pain behavior — can be defined with very little accuracy, primarily because it is a problem caused by a multitude of factors: fitness, job, education, financial consequences of disability, and most important, personal choice.

The fact is that in many severely disabled people, organic pathology is minimal. This situation frustrates patient, physician, and insuring agency. And it often leads to an endless and unrewarding search for a cause that cannot be found.

Hippocrates said: "Look not at the disease in the person; look at the person with the disease." Since ancient times, doctors have been exhorted to recognize that disease occurs as but one variable in a complex multitude of factors which can dwarf the existing organic pathology.

A major factor in exacerbating disability is well-meaning but inappropriate compensation benefits. When the financial, social, and job factors are all added up, being disabled can, for some, be more attractive and rewarding in the short term than taking a positive approach and struggling to improve the situation. A balanced compensation policy should reward people who struggle to prove ability and combat loss; it should not reward those who fail to do so. Compensation policies that give pensions for *minor or nonexisting* organic pathology or for pain alone hurt society as a whole and beggar the patient in particular.

The compensation situation usually becomes "terminally pathological" when the patient engages a lawyer. In our society, whenever something goes wrong, we look around for someone to *blame*. "Someone's at fault." "Someone will be made to pay." "It wasn't my fault."

There is no question that individuals in our society who have suffered wrong or loss should be compensated. We ask only if the balance has shifted too far, so that disability is encouraged or even rewarded. When invalid behavior — disability — becomes fully established over time, restoration to full function is rare, even in an individual with minimal organic pathology. It is one more example of a self-fulfilling prophecy.

A system that fosters the development of disability is a system in need of appraisal and change. Consider these factors:
- a tendency in the compensation system to reward the complainer and ignore the stoic;
- an emphasis in the political system on funding for *disease* (98 percent of funds), not for prevention (2 percent of funds);
- a custom in the legal system to blame "someone. . . anyone" but assume no risk for the plaintiff;
- a tradition in the health system to treat disease but place little emphasis on personal control, on prevention, and on freedom of choice.

The sum total is a situation where the simple has become complex; where high-tech solutions are sought for low-tech problems; and where common-sense initiatives have been lost in a sea of bureaucracy.

Indeed, these and other factors in our compensation system cry out for fresh appraisal and change.

A Personal Challenge

For thousands of years, humankind's innate sense was to scrounge for enough food to eat in order to survive. Now survival can mean learning how to deal with plenty, in every sense of the word. In terms of food, we now see diseases that can be traced to excess intake.

We have in many ways reached a pinnacle of human achievement. We are programmed to take the labor out of work, to make the sweat of our brows easier. Now the challenge is to use our bodies enough to keep sedentary diseases away.

We have learned to control many risks in our environment, from floods to epidemics. Now the challenge is to deal with the personal risks in ourselves.

With Back Power, we offer you a manual to help you manage your own personal back risks. And with it, this challenge: *Do you dare to be the best you can be?*

Index